Quick Reference

Abusive
Head Trauma

*for Health Care Professionals,
Social Services, and Law Enforcement*

W0232393

G.W. Medical Publishing, Inc.
St. Louis
www.gwmedical.com

i

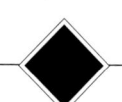

Contents in Brief

Quick Reference
Abusive
Head Trauma

for Health Care Professionals,
Social Services, and Law Enforcement

Lori D. Frasier, MD, FAAP
Associate Professor of Pediatrics
University of Utah School of Medicine
Medical Director, Medical Assessment Team
Center for Safe and Healthy Families
Primary Children's Medical Center
Salt Lake City, Utah

Kay Rauth-Farley, MD, FAAP
Clinical Assistant Professor
Department of Pediatrics
School of Medicine
University of Kansas Medical Center
Kansas City, Kansas
Medical Director
Sunflower House Children's Advocacy Center
Shawnee, Kansas

Randell Alexander, MD, PhD, FAAP
Professor of Pediatrics, and Chief
Division of Child Protection and Forensic Pediatrics
Department of Pediatrics
University of Florida
Jacksonville, Florida
Statewide Medical Director, Florida Child Protection Teams
Children's Medical Services
Professor of Pediatrics
Morehouse School of Medicine
Atlanta, Georgia

Robert N. Parrish, JD
Managing Attorney
Second District Office of the Guardian ad Litem
Layton, Utah

G.W. Medical Publishing, Inc.
St. Louis
www.gwmedical.com

Publishers: Glenn E. Whaley and Marianne V. Whaley
Art Director: Glenn E. Whaley
Managing Editors: Megan O. Hayes
                 Karen C. Maurer
Associate Editors: Christine M. Bauer
                 Robert J. Lewis
                 Sandi Villarreal
Book Design/Page Layout: G.W. Graphics
                 Sudon Choe
                 Charles J. Seibel, III
Print/Production Coordinator: Charles J. Seibel, III
Cover Design: G.W. Graphics
Color Prepress Specialist: Charles J. Seibel, III
Developmental Editor: Elaine Steinborn
Copy Editor: Sheri Kubasek
Proofreader: Michael S. McConnell
Indexer: Robert A. Saigh

Printed in Canada

Publisher:
G.W. Medical Publishing, Inc.
77 Westport Plaza, Suite 366, St. Louis, Missouri 63146-3124 USA
Phone: (314)542-4213 Fax: (314)542-4239 Toll Free: (800)600-0330
http://www.gwmedical.com

Library of Congress Cataloging-in-Publication Data

Abusive head trauma quick reference : for health care professionals, social services, and law enforcement / [edited by] Lori D. Frasier ... [et al.].
     p. ; cm.
  Abbreviated version of: Abusive head trauma in infants and children / Lori Frasier ... [et al.]. c2006.
  Includes bibliographical references and index.
  ISBN-13: 978-1-878060-57-0
  ISBN-10: 1-878060-57-0
  1. Child abuse--Handbooks, manuals, etc. 2. Head--Wounds and injuries--Handbooks, manuals, etc. I. Frasier, Lori, 1955- II. Abusive head trauma in infants and children.
  [DNLM: 1. Child Abuse--diagnosis--Handbooks. 2. Craniocerebral Trauma--Handbooks.
    3. Child Abuse--legislation & jurisprudence--Handbooks. 4. Child Abuse--prevention & control--Handbooks. 5. Child. 6. Infant. WL 39 A167 2007]
  RJ1122.5.A2889 2007
  616.85'8223--dc22
                     2007008146

CONTRIBUTORS

Marilyn Barr, BIS, SSW
Founder and Executive Director
National Center on Shaken Baby Syndrome
Ogden, Utah, USA
Director
BC Shaken Baby Syndrome Prevention
Programme
Vancouver, BC, Canada

Ronald G. Barr, MDCM, FRCPC
Professor of Pediatrics
University of British Columbia Faculty of
Medicine
Canada Research Chair in Community Child
Health Research
Director
Center for Community Child Health Research,
Child and Family Research Institute
BC Children's Hospital
Vancouver, BC, Canada

Scott A. Benton, MD, FAAP
Director of Pediatric Forensic Medicine
Clinical Associate Professor of Pediatrics
LSU & Tulane Departments of Pediatrics
Audrey Hepburn Children At Risk Evaluation
(CARE) Center
Children's Hospital
New Orleans, Louisiana

Gail V. Benton, DDS
Clinical Assistant Professor of Pediatric
Dentistry
LSU School of Dentistry
Audrey Hepburn Children At Risk Evaluation
(CARE) Center
Children's Hospital
New Orleans, Louisiana

Bradford W. Betz, MD, MS
Advanced Radiology Services, PC
Grand Rapids, Michigan
Medical Director, Department of Radiology
DeVos Children's Hospital
Grand Rapids, Michigan
Associate Clinical Professor of Radiology
Michigan State University
East Lansing, Michigan

Stephen C. Boos, MD, FAAP
Associate Professor of Clinical Pediatrics
University of Medicine and Dentistry of New
Jersey
School of Osteopathic Medicine
New Jersey Cares Institute
Stratford, New Jersey
Medical Director
Treehouse, Child Assessment Center of
Montgomery County
Rockville, Montgomery County, Maryland

Julie Bradshaw, LCSW
Director
Primary Children's Center for Safe and Healthy
Families
Primary Children's Medical Center
Salt Lake City, Utah

Marguerite M. Caré, MD
Assistant Professor of Pediatric Radiology
Division of Neuroradiology
Cincinnati Children's Hospital Medical Center
Cincinnati, Ohio

Karen Coleman
Marketing and Development Coordinator
Prevent Child Abuse Utah
Ogden, Utah

M. Denise Dowd, MD, MPH
Professor of Pediatrics
Children's Mercy Hospital
University of Missouri-Kansas City
Kansas City, Missouri

Detective Bruce Foremny
Glendale Police Department (retired)
Criminal Investigator
Arizona Department of Juvenile Corrections
Bruce Foremny Consulting, LLC
Litchfield Park, Arizona

Todd C. Grey, MD
Chief Medical Examiner
State of Utah
Adjunct Associate Professor of Pathology
University of Utah School of Medicine
Salt Lake City, Utah

Sam P. Gulino, MD
Assistant Professor of Pathology and Laboratory
Medicine
University of South Florida College of
Medicine
Deputy Chief Medical Examiner
Hillsborough County Medical Examiner
Department
Tampa, Florida

Karen Kirhofer Hansen, MD
Associate Professor of Pediatrics
University of Utah
Pediatrician, Safe and Healthy Families Team
Primary Children's Medical Center
Salt Lake City, Utah

Gary L. Hedlund, DO
Associate Professor of Radiology
University of Utah School of Medicine
Pediatric Neuroradiologist
Chairman, Department of Medical Imaging
Primary Children's Medical Center
Salt Lake City, Utah

Robert O. Hoffman, MD
Associate Professor of Ophthalmology
Director, Pediatric Ophthalmology Division
Department of Ophthalmology and Visual
Sciences
University of Utah College of Medicine
Chairman of Ophthalmology
Primary Children's Medical Center
Salt Lake City, Utah

Peter Kan, MD
Resident, Neurosurgery
Department of Neurosurgery
University of Utah
Salt Lake City, Utah

James R. Lauridson, MD
Chief Medical Examiner
Alabama Department of Forensic Sciences
Nibbana Graphics, LLC
Montgomery, Alabama

Deborah E. Lowen, MD, FAAP
Assistant Professor of Pediatrics
University of Oklahoma College of Medicine -
Tulsa
Medical Director, Children's JUSTICE Center
Tulsa, Oklahoma

Nick Mamalis, MD
Professor of Ophthalmology
Director of Ophthalmic Pathology
John Moran Eye Center
University of Utah
Salt Lake City, Utah

Wayne I. Munkel, MSW, LCSW
Supervisor, Social Services
SSM Cardinal Glennon Children's Medical
Center
St. Louis, Missouri
Co-Chair Missouri Child Fatality Review Panel
State of Missouri
Jefferson City, Missouri

Vincent J. Palusci, MD, MS
Helppie Endowed Professor of Pediatrics
Wayne State University School of Medicine
Medical Director, Child Protection Center
Children's Hospital of Michigan
Detroit, Michigan

Michael D. Partington, MD, FACS, FAAP
Pediatric Neurosurgery
Gillette Children's Specialty Healthcare and
Children's Hospitals and Clinics of Minnesota
Saint Paul, Minnesota

Leslie K. Pfeil, BSN, RN, CCRN(P)
Charge Nurse, Urgent Care Center
Children's Mercy South
Overland Park, Kansas
Staff Nurse, Pediatric Intensive Care Unit
Children At Risk Team
Children's Mercy Hospital
Kansas City, Missouri

Gregory A. Schmunk, MD, FACP, FASCP
Forensic Pathologist
Polk County Medical Examiner
Des Moines, Iowa

Andrew Sirotnak, MD
Associate Professor of Pediatrics
University of Colorado School of Medicine
Director, Kempe Child Protection Team
The Children's Hospital
Kempe Center for the Prevention and
Treatment of Child Abuse & Neglect
Denver, Colorado

Betty Spivack, MD
Assistant Professor of Pediatrics and Pathology
University of Louisville School of Medicine
Louisville, Kentucky
Co-Director, Clinical Forensic Program
Division of Forensic Pathology and Clinical
Forensic Medicine
University of Louisville School of Medicine
Department of Pathology
Louisville, Kentucky

David A. Start, MD
Forensic Pathologist
Spectrum Health—Blodgett Campus
Department of Pathology
Medical Examiner
Kent and Ottawa County
Grand Rapids, Michigan

Trina Taylor, BS, SSW
Prevent Child Abuse Utah
Ogden, Utah

Marion L. Walker, MD
Professor of Neurological Surgery
Chairman, Division of Pediatric Neurosurgery
University of Utah
Primary Children's Medical Center
Salt Lake City, Utah

Amy Wicks
SBS Information and Research Specialist
National Center on Shaken Baby Syndrome
Ogden, Utah

Debra Williams, BS
Research Specialist
SBS Hospital Education Program Coordinator
National Center on Shaken Baby Syndrome
Ogden, Utah

FOREWORD

The existence of "shaken baby syndrome" (the triad of signs consisting of unexplained encephalopathy, subdural hemorrhages, and retinal hemorrhages) has been widely debated. Sometimes it is difficult to tell if a child's head has been shaken, impacted, or crushed; whether the blood supply to the brain was purposefully occluded; or if another event may have caused a healthy, happy child to become suddenly ill with serious head trauma. The editors of this book have recognized this difficulty and adopted the term "abusive head trauma" (AHT) instead. This term conveys the understanding that the previously healthy child suffered an inflicted injury, but the mechanism of injury—of which shaking is merely one—is not presumed.

Abusive Head Trauma Quick Reference breaks new ground in many ways. First, it is comprehensive in its approach. Every aspect of AHT is covered, from neuroscience to prosecution. This text is truly multidisciplinary, involving health professionals, law enforcement officers, legal prosecutors, social welfare experts, mental health professionals, and rehabilitation specialists.

Another exciting aspect of this book is that a new generation of experts is writing exciting chapters. The list of authors demonstrates that the field is expanding and vigorous. Many new people have acquired expertise in diagnosing and treating abusive head trauma. It is refreshing to see a child abuse text that highlights the work of new experts. Although the ancestry of this book can be traced to the work of John Caffey, C. Henry Kempe, Ray E. Helfer, Norman Guthkelch, and other legends in the field, it is clear that the field is in competent hands with the current generation.

The subject of AHT is approached with a critical eye on literature and extensive clinical experience, providing the readers with balanced sources of data. Finally, the case-based approach makes this text an excellent resource for teachers of medicine and related disciplines as well as for "life-long learners" who want to sharpen their diagnostic acumen and medical skills.

The field of child abuse medicine has come a long way in a short time. This book is yet another landmark on our road to understanding the infant brain and its unique vulnerabilities. I thank the editors and authors for documenting our progress thus far.

Carole Jenny, MD, MBA
Professor of Pediatrics
Brown Medical School
Director, ChildSafe Child Protection Program
Hasbro Children's Hospital
Providence, Rhode Island

FOREWORD

Today's courtrooms have become the battleground for lawyers and experts who challenge the core science of medical research and theory on abusive head trauma (AHT). It is a battle fought before jurors and judges who have little knowledge of the scientific and medical issues that they are supposed to determine. Amidst this chaotic battle sits the judicial system and its search for truth and justice; however, the end result in many instances is confusion, deception, and a loss of integrity in both the science and the law—a sad and tragic epilogue in the wake of the even more significant loss or destruction of a small and precious human life.

For those involved in responding to child maltreatment, these stories occur far too frequently. Few professionals exposed to these scenarios question the reality that children are the daily victims of violent acts perpetrated by those who are supposed to love and protect them the most. For professionals, it is not a question of understanding and believing that these situations exist, but instead of getting others to understand these same truths and to explain why these truths should be accepted. This is no easy task.

The last two decades have witnessed an unprecedented growth in the state of medical research and knowledge regarding AHT. This increased knowledge base has brought with it improvements in the recognition and diagnosis of such trauma by medical professionals, concomitant increases in referrals of these findings to other investigating and prosecuting agencies, and more frequent legal filings through both the juvenile and criminal courts. If there is one thing we have learned from the trials, tribulations, and controversies of the past, it is that a multidisciplinary, coordinated response to these cases is the most effective method for coordinating information, promoting knowledge, improving professional practice, and arriving at the truth. The multidisciplinary nature of *Abusive Head Trauma Quick Reference* reflects the importance of this principle and the value of this approach.

The educational value of this text is to be found not only in alerting professionals to the current issues and controversies that we all face, but also as a compilation of current professional thought against which novel and controversial theories can be tested and judged. Readers will be encouraged to elevate their own practice to the standards outlined by these experts, and perhaps as importantly, they will be motivated to seek additional knowledge from professionals both within and without their fields of practice. All should be challenged to develop best practices for themselves and their communities. No lesser standards can hope to withstand the rigors of the current and future challenges that are meted out in the crucible of the courtroom.

Brian Holmgren

Assistant District Attorney General
Davidson County District Attorney Generals Office
Nashville, Tennessee

FOREWORD

From 2000 to 2004, I was charged with the responsibility of advising police officers in the United Kingdom on how to investigate cases of child abuse. In doing so, I gained unique insight into how the many professionals involved in investigating and treating these cases actually carry out their work. I have been lucky to work with truly committed doctors, nurses, forensic pathologists, lawyers, and social service workers in countries such as Sweden, the United States, Canada, Bermuda, Germany, Estonia, and the United Kingdom. It has been my privilege to work with and learn from many of the professionals who have given their time to this book.

Every year, in countries all over the world, children are injured or killed as a result of abusive head trauma. During the last few years, the nomenclature for describing these injuries has changed from Caffey's "whiplash shaken infant syndrome" of the 1970s to the "shaken baby syndrome" of the 1990s. The title of this reference work, *Abusive Head Trauma*, more accurately reflects the true nature of how these children are injured and killed.

When I researched abusive head trauma (AHT) on behalf of the Home Office from 2000 to 2003, I was surprised to find a lack of reference works on this extremely important issue. That gap is now being addressed, and these new publications are written for both professionals and the public. This book is the first illustrated clinical and photographic quick reference on AHT, and it will be invaluable to all disciplines involved in child abuse cases. Only by working in a truly multidisciplinary environment can we hope to understand these cases and build strategies to treat, investigate, and prevent them.

This book does exactly that by addressing medical, legal, nursing, social service, and investigative issues of AHT. What it cannot do is show the grief and despair encountered by parents who have lost a child to AHT or soothe a young victim. The professionals who have contributed to this book have encountered that grief and despair many times, and it is one of the driving factors as to why they have given their time and energy to helping educate colleagues and public alike.

The dedication shown by all professionals working in this arena is clear. Thank you for your efforts, on behalf of injured and abused children everywhere, in bringing this book to fruition.

Philip L. Wheeler

Detective Chief Inspector
Central Operations
New Scotland Yard
London, England

PREFACE

In the last decade, as more communities have worked to develop effective methods for recognizing and treating victims, investigating cases, protecting victims from further harm, prosecuting offenders, and pursuing education and prevention efforts, there has been a growing interest in educating and training the professionals involved in all phases of the community's response to this problem. It is time to share information in an organized, comprehensive, and useful manner among professionals working in the field in order to provide improved recognition, treatment, investigation, prosecution, education, and prevention of this deadly form of abuse.

This text, which is an abbreviated version of the primary reference *Abusive Head Trauma in Infants and Children*, is designed to serve as an easy-to-use field reference for medical, investigative, legal, social service, and prevention professionals. All of these disciplines are affected by abusive head trauma (AHT) in children and all have made notable progress in handling the results of child maltreatment in general. The goal of educating all professionals is to help children and families with the corollary of improving society's concern and care for the most helpless of its citizens.

The chapters offered here attempt to put the problem in perspective with respect to current attitudes and practices. In addition, notable differences between accidental brain injury and AHT are discussed in terms of the mechanisms of injury and the other signs to observe. Special considerations for the areas of nursing, radiology, neuroradiology, neurosurgery, and ophthalmology are addressed in specific chapters. Disorders that mimic AHT and fall into the differential diagnosis are carefully explained. As with other types of child maltreatment, the occurrence of associated injuries can help in making an accurate diagnosis, so the specific findings that distinguish AHT from other causes of injury are discussed in detail.

Specialists serving in social service, forensic, and prosecutorial roles will find chapters covering the contributions they make to resolving cases of AHT. The latest courtroom aids are explained to help present an accurate and visually compelling case. The roles of individuals who come into contact with children suffering from AHT are detailed to provide the background needed to deal with cases expeditiously. Each chapter emphasizes caring for the child and family as well as identifying the problem and the perpetrator.

We have sought to offer a balanced approach to the problem of AHT while exploring current efforts and recommendations to address the concerns of professionals. It is hoped that this publication will become a reliable field reference for professionals in the medical, investigative, legal, social service, and prevention areas.

Lori Frasier, MD, FAAP

Kay Rauth-Farley, MD, FAAP

Randell Alexander, MD, PhD, FAAP

Robert N. Parrish, JD

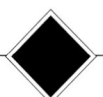

CONTENTS IN DETAIL

CHAPTER 7: MEDICAL DISORDERS THAT MIMIC ABUSIVE HEAD TRAUMA

CHAPTER 8: NURSING CARE

CHAPTER 11: FORENSIC INVESTIGATIONS

Quick Reference

Abusive
Head Trauma

*for Health Care Professionals,
Social Services, and Law Enforcement*

G.W. Medical Publishing, Inc.
St. Louis
www.gwmedical.com

Chapter 1

RECOGNIZING INTENTIONAL AND UNINTENTIONAL HEAD INJURIES

Stephen C. Boos, MD, FAAP
M. Denise Dowd, MD, MPH
Kay Rauth-Farley, MD, FAAP
Lori D. Frasier, MD, FAAP
Todd C. Grey, MD
Robert N. Parrish, JD

INCIDENCE

— Each year in the United States approximately 100 of every 100 000 children younger than 6 years suffer traumatic brain injuries causing death or hospitalization[1]; 82% of cases are mild and 5% are fatal.

— Leading mechanisms and annual rates of head injuries[1]:

1. Falls: 50.6 per 100 000 children.

2. Motor vehicle crashes: 25.9 per 100 000 children.

3. Abuse: 12.8 per 100 000 children.

— Severe accidental injuries are rarely seen in infants younger than 1 year.[2]

— Most head injuries in children aged 1 year and older are unintentional (**Figures 1-1-a** to **f**).

— Accidental head injuries are more common in boys and frequently occur in the spring and summer months and on weekends, when children are most active (**Figures 1-2-a** to **c**).

— Certain medical disorders (hydrocephalus with a shunt and co-agulation disorders such as hemophilia and vitamin K deficiency) increase the risk for intracranial injuries with less force.

— Intracranial injuries:

1. Are significantly more common in abusive than in unintentional injuries.[3]

2. Differ in the frequencies of specific types.

    A. Subdural hematomas (SDHs): 10% unintentional, 46% abusive.

    B. Subarachnoid hemorrhages (SAHs): 8% unintentional, 31% abusive.[4]

— Epidural hematomas (EDH) are more common with unintentional head trauma than with abusive head trauma (AHT).

— AHT describes circumstances surrounding head injuries but does not limit the scope of the mechanisms involved in producing injury.

— Serious head injuries are usually caused by abuse.

— It is necessary to understand the mechanism of injury for each type of physical finding.

COMMON MECHANISMS OF UNINTENTIONAL HEAD INJURY

— General categories include direct contact with the head, acceleration or deceleration of the brain within the skull, and hypoxia-ischemia.

— Several mechanisms can be combined.

— Most severe unintentional head injuries are accompanied by a notable injury history.

FALLS

— Falls down stairs rarely cause serious intracranial injury, except when children are in baby walkers.

1. This includes the initial fall and any subsequent short falls.

2. Physical damage is caused by the cumulative effect of kinetic energy.

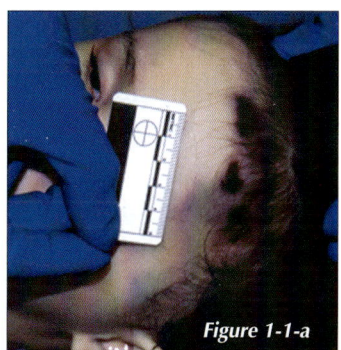
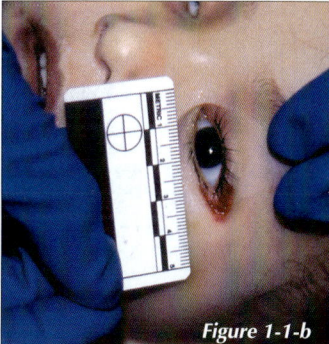

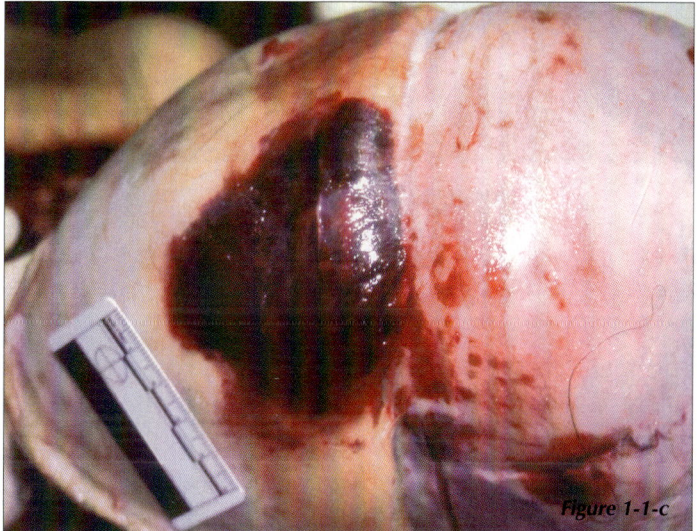

***Figures 1-1-a** to **f.** Two-year-old girl crushed by a 27-inch television. She suffered an irregular abrasion to the left forehead (a); a small laceration at the lateral corner of the left eye (b); scalp and subgaleal contusions in the left frontal and inferior occipital regions (c); transverse linear skull fracture (d and e); and right occipital subdural hematoma with irregular subarachnoid hemorrhage in the right occipital and left frontal regions, cortical contusions of the right occipital pole, and cerebral edema with herniation (f).*

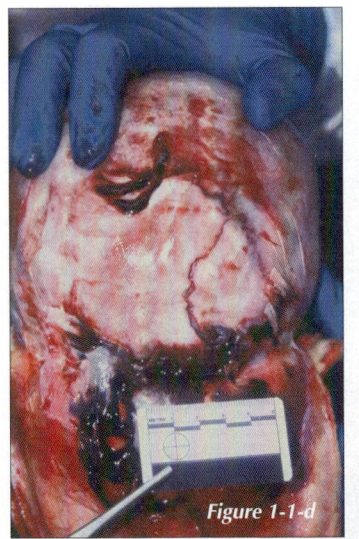

Figure 1-1-d

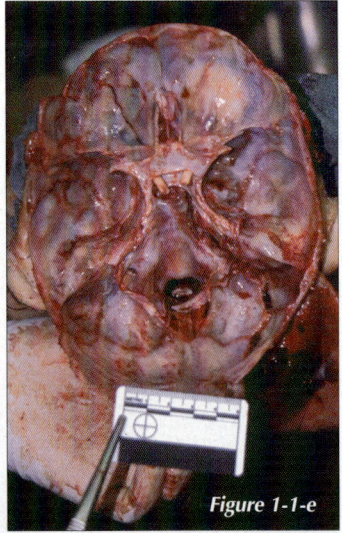

Figure 1-1-e

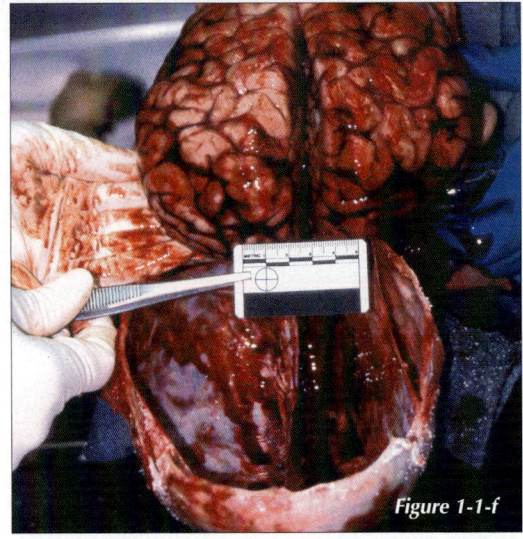

Figure 1-1-f

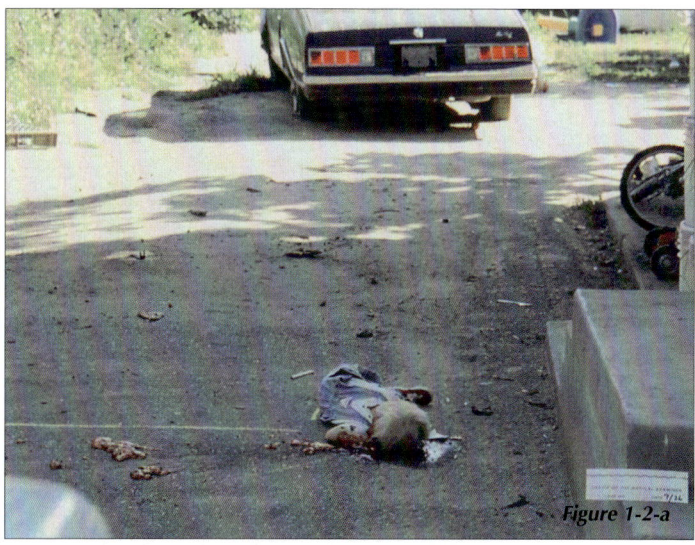

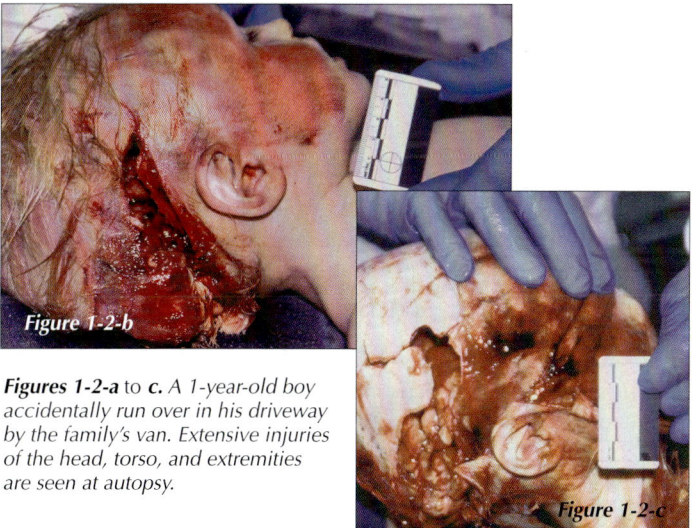

Figures 1-2-a to **c.** *A 1-year-old boy accidentally run over in his driveway by the family's van. Extensive injuries of the head, torso, and extremities are seen at autopsy.*

3.   There is no correlation between injury severity and number of stairs.

4.   Risk of skull fracture in baby walker falls depends on the number of steps and whether the head strikes a concrete floor.

— Depressed skull fractures are uncommon and generally occur only in short, witnessed falls in which children fall against a hard edge.[5]

— EDHs are rare but possible, especially with a direct blow to the parietal skull overlying the middle meningeal artery.

— SDHs are only seen in falls greater than 1.22 m (4 ft).[6]

— Complex skull fractures, including depressed and basilar or bilateral skull fractures, are more likely in falls from heights greater than 1.22 m (4 ft) and falls down stairs.

— The following are factors used to determine the minimum height at which severe head injuries can occur in a fall.

1.   *Fall data.* Distance fallen, resistance of the surface fallen onto, rotational forces, whether the fall is broken, whether the child hits another object on the way down, and whether the child was in motion or propelled before hitting the surface.

2.   *Age of child.* Younger skulls are more elastic and resistant to skull fractures.

3.   *History.* Often false in AHT.

MOTOR VEHICLE CRASHES

— Crashes cause the most severe unintentional childhood head injuries (**Figures 1-3-a** to **e**).

— Head injuries are related to acceleration-deceleration mechanisms or direct contact of the head with fixed objects in the car.

— Injuries are similar to those seen with shaking or shaking/impact (subdural and epidural hematomas, brain contusions, and diffuse axonal injuries).

— Secondary injuries are from shock.

— Ejection from the car greatly increases the potential for severe, often fatal, brain injury.

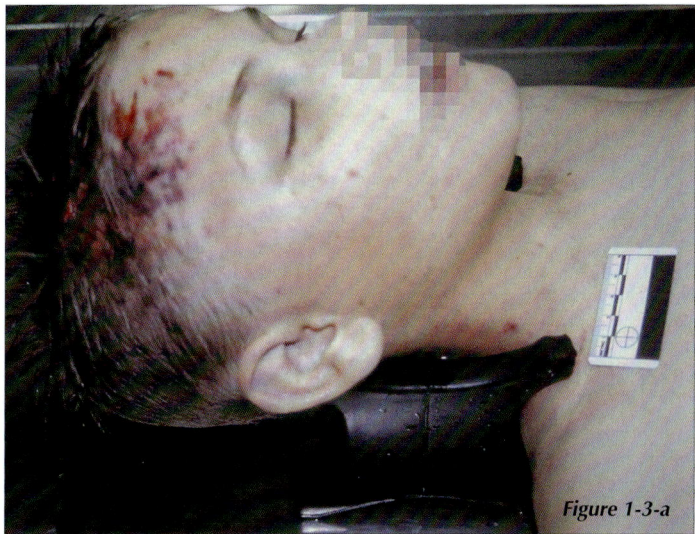

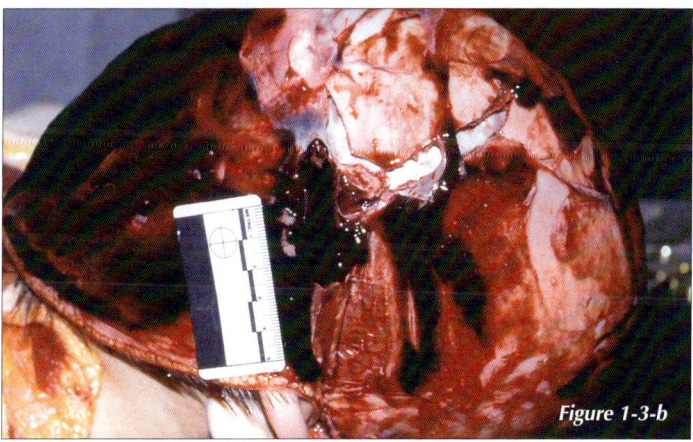

Figure 1-3-a. *Abrasion and contusion of the right frontotemporal region on boy unintentionally killed in a motor vehicle crash.*

Figure 1-3-b. *Extensive subgaleal contusion.*

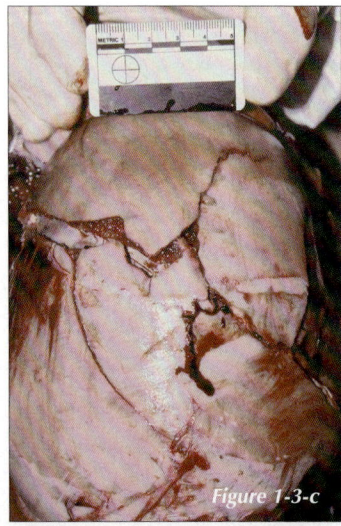

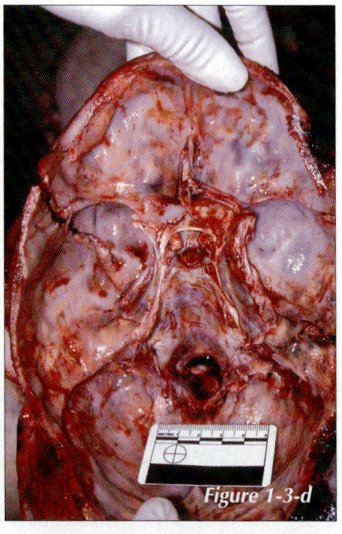

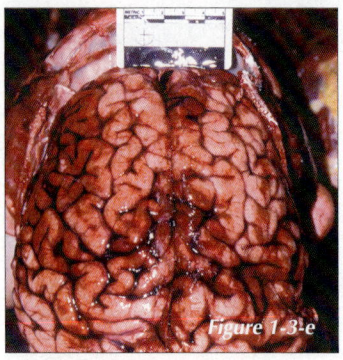

Figures 1-3-c and **d.** Complex fracturing of the vault and base of the skull.

Figure 1-3-e. Thin subdural hematoma with subarachnoid hemorrhage over the convexities and cerebral edema.

PLAYGROUND INJURIES

— Head injuries are the second most common type of injury sustained on playgrounds,[7] but most are minor and caused by falls.

— Severity depends on the height of the fall and the landing surface.

1. Playground surfaces with greater shock-absorbing ability (eg, rub-

berized surfaces or those covered with at least 12 inches of loose fill such as pea gravel or wood chips) are less likely to be associated with severe head injuries.

2. Compact, firm surfaces (eg, concrete, asphalt, grass, dirt) increase head injury risk and are not recommended for playgrounds.

DIFFERENTIATING ABUSIVE FROM UNINTENTIONAL HEAD INJURY
— Collect and document history and physical examination.

1. Examination must match history.

2. AHT is often accompanied by other injuries.

3. A depressed neurological state can complicate finding concomitant injuries.

4. **Table 1-1** lists indicators of abuse.

TASKS FOR PHYSICIANS (**Table 1-2**)
— Recognize patterns suspicious for abuse.

— Obtain the full clinical picture, including historical and physical clues.

— Identify causes of ailments.

— Develop an objective assessment of the nature, severity, and timing of the trauma.

— Help authorities understand the significance and limitations of information so they can best determine whether children were abused, who might be responsible, and how recurrences can be prevented.

PATTERNS SUGGESTING ABUSE
See **Table 1-3**.

SHAKEN BABY SYNDROME
Typical Characteristics
— A typical case involves an infant younger than 1 year brought to the emergency department with sudden onset of unconsciousness and respiratory irregularities or seizure.

Table 1-1. Possible Indicators of Abuse

— Coexisting injuries that cannot be explained

— Delayed action of caregiver in seeking medical attention of child

— History of how the injury occurred that is inconsistent with the injury

— Proposed mechanism of injury inconsistent with the child's developmental capability

— History that another child inflicted the injury

— History of injury that changes between caregivers and/or over time

Table 1-2. Tasks for Physicians

— Recognize patterns that suggest possible child abuse

— Elucidate all pertinent historical, examination, laboratory, and imaging findings

— Identify alternative medical explanations or recognize traumatic etiology

— Reach a sound assessment of the nature, severity, and timing of trauma

— If history does not provide for innocent explanatory trauma, work with appropriate agencies to establish abuse and identify abusers

Table 1-3. Patterns Suggesting Abuse

— Shaken baby syndrome (SBS)

— Variants of SBS, such as shaken impact syndrome

— Battered child syndrome

— Mild and misdiagnosed abusive head trauma

— Trauma with absent or inconsistent history

— The history provided suggests sudden, unprovoked symptoms.

— The physical examination shows serious illness but no external evidence of trauma.

— Computed tomography (CT) scan shows SDH and diffuse parenchymal injury with edema and cerebral swelling.

— Occult trauma and possible child abuse are recognized; additional studies are performed.

1. Skeletal radiographs show old fractures of posterior ribs and metaphyseal ends of long bones.

2. On dilated indirect ophthalmoscopy, extensive retinal hemorrhages involving multiple layers are found in both eyes.

— The infant commonly requires mechanical ventilation and measures to control increased intracranial pressure.

— Coma usually remits after several days and life support is discontinued, but severe neurodevelopmental handicaps result.[8]

Variations in History and Physical Findings
— The average age of victims is 3 to 10 months, but shaken baby syndrome can be seen in children as old as 3 years.

— Infants are often reported to have fallen from couches, beds, etc.

— Adults may describe shaking infants during play or when trying to revive them after the onset of unprovoked symptoms.

— The force of shaking is often minimized until inconsistencies in the history are noted, then the reported level of force increases but innocent intent is maintained.

— Histories change as guilty adults try to fabricate explanations.[9]

— External evidence of head impact and old or new trauma may be found on the body.[10]

— Rib and/or metaphyseal fractures are lacking in 38% to 65% of cases.[4,9]

— Whether severe or mild, symptomatic or asymptomatic, head injuries must be accompanied by a history that includes explanatory trauma. Inconsistencies may be seen in biomechanics, epidemiology, temporal issues, and developmental abilities.

BATTERED CHILD SYNDROME

— Involves the co-occurrence of multiple injuries from distinct and inadequately explained traumatic causes.

— The syndrome can accompany AHT.

— Inflicted trauma in the home is the most likely cause.[11]

— Evidence of old head injuries can be found in 30% to 50% of AHT cases.[12-14]

— Look for skeletal injuries that show evidence of healing, scars, or reports of earlier cutaneous injuries.

— The chance of abusive injury increases with repeated unexplained traumatic injuries.

— The more varied the forms of repeated trauma, the less likely they are to be explained by an underlying medical condition.

MILD AHT

— Findings include acute SDHs but no parenchymal brain injuries, retinal hemorrhages, fractures, or other evidence of abuse.

— Traumatic cause is evident. If the history does not mention trauma or reports trauma inconsistent with the findings, suspect abusive injury.

— A small number of cases have no identifiable cause.

— Maintain reasonable concern for inflicted injuries when assessing children with chronic SDHs.

— Moderately severe intracranial injuries (eg, cerebral contusions and small SDHs) may result from longer falls (ie, from bunk beds, down stairs).[15-17]

1. If no history of trauma is given, abuse is likely.

2. With multiple, depressed, branched, or diastatic skull fractures,

multiple, focused, or more severe impacts are expected.[18-20]

— Factors involved in the misdiagnosis of AHT:

1.   AHT may be overlooked in children from white, traditional families and in children with milder symptoms, such as fussiness, mild lethargy, and vomiting.

2.   Young infants rarely have bruising of the head, especially when they cannot stand alone,[21] so the presence of head or facial bruises in infants with neurological changes or vomiting without diarrhea should prompt the search for traumatic cause.

3.   It is not reasonable to obtain CT scans of all children with fussiness, mild lethargy, or vomiting without diarrhea. However, finding these symptoms in infants with other mild indications of trauma is a pattern that should raise concern for abuse, regardless of the family's social situation.

THE EXAMINATION

SUBJECTIVE ASSESSMENT

— Stabilize the child's condition.

— Note patterns suggesting AHT.

— Set aside significant time to interview adults involved.

1.   Begin with open-ended, unstructured questions.

2.   Ask for increasingly specific details.

3.   Determine the last time when the child was clearly normal.

4.   Ask for specific explanations for each injury.

5.   Carefully record the information.

— Coordinate further questioning with investigative agencies. This step is often handled by child protective services (CPS) or law enforcement personnel.

1.   Note inconsistencies between the histories given and the child's condition.

2.   Ask direct questions based on how you believe the child was injured.

— Obtain past history, family history, social history, and review of systems.

1. *Past history.* Birth events, past medical illnesses, preceding neurological complaints, earlier incidences of trauma, physical growth, developmental course, and current abilities.

2. *Family history.* Inherited conditions (metabolic disorders), unexplained mental retardation, fetal loss (suggesting undiagnosed metabolic disorders), bleeding disorders, osteogenesis imperfecta, and nonhereditary family data such as the presence of domestic violence and substance abuse and past involvement with CPS or law enforcement.

3. *Social situation.* Financial and other stressors; who has unsupervised access to the child.

— May inquire whether families believe children could have been abused.

— May inform families of suspected abuse. Such forewarning may not be favored by law enforcement officers or prosecutors.

— Collect as much medical history as possible before police and social services personnel begin investigations (**Table 1-4**).

Table 1-4. Subjective Assessment: Interview Each Caregiver Separately
— Unstructured request for explanation
— Specific request for explanation of identified trauma
— Past medical history, including birth, illnesses, neurological complaints, trauma, and growth and development
— Family history of heritable medical conditions
— Family history of violence, substance use, and past agency involvement
— Family stressors, family composition, and people with access to the child
— Review of systems
— Coordination with agencies to confront each historian with inconsistencies

OBJECTIVE ASSESSMENT
— Assess temperature and head circumference.

1. Fever may be caused by bleeding in the head, infection, or AHT.

2. Hypothermia is a sign of delay in seeking medical care.[22]

3. An especially large head circumference, added to abnormal development and dystonia, may indicate glutaricaciduria type I, which can manifest as acute unexplained SDHs.[23]

4. In chronic SDHs, seek marked increases in growth velocity of the head to determine when the original trauma occurred (**Table 1-5**).

Table 1-5. Objective Assessment

— Complete physical examination
— Detailed examination of head, face, neck, ears, oral cavity, skin surfaces, genitals, and anus
— Acute head CT scan
— Delayed head MRI scan
— Skeletal radiograph survey, acute and in 2 weeks
— Abdominal CT scan if unresponsive, multiple trauma, or indicated by laboratory tests
— Laboratory tests: CBC, PT/INR, PTT, basic chemistry panel, AST, ALT, amylase, urinalysis; consider serial testing
— Dilated indirect ophthalmoscopy by an ophthalmologist

Head, Eye, Ear, Nose, and Throat
— Thoroughly inspect and palpate the scalp.

— Note bruises, contusions, abrasions, and lacerations; they are evidence of head impact.

— Palpate for bogginess or swelling.

1. Swelling may be the only evidence of recent injury.

2. Absence of swelling over a skull fracture may indicate passage of time.[24]

— Hemotympanum on otoscopic examination may indicate possible basilar skull fractures.

— Observe for fine petechiae in curls of the pinna and hematomas on the edge or behind the pinna. Petechiae occur in child abuse but rarely accidentally.[25]

— Subconjunctival hemorrhages or petechiae indicate direct trauma or strangulation.

— Retinal hemorrhages on direct ophthalmoscopy are strong evidence of AHT. Dilated indirect ophthalmoscopy examinations by ophthalmologists can better determine specificity.[26] See Chapter 5, Ophthalmology.

— Note any injury or dried blood in the mouth or nose indicating direct injury.

1. Observe the oral surface of the lips and frenulae of the tongue and lips.

2. Tears of the labial frenulum and contusions inside lips suggest blows to the mouth or suffocation injuries.

3. Tears of the lingual frenulum occur when objects are forced into the mouth, suggesting violence and events leading to AHT.

Neck

— Internal injuries of the neck are found in fatal AHT but are seldom found in living patients.[27-30]

— Note external neck injuries.

1. If the child is in an immobilization collar, remove it so the entire surface of the neck can be seen.

2. Look for cutaneous lesions over carotid arteries.

3. Note bruising, abrasions, induration, or local redness, indicating strangulation.

4.   Ligature marks are very rare.

5.   Palpate the posterior neck.

6.   Perform radiological assessment of the cervical spine.

Skin

— Evaluate all skin surfaces in detail.

— Severely injured children are typically placed on their backs. Once stabilized, roll them from side to side to assess the back and buttocks.

— Note new bruises, contusions, abrasions, lacerations, incisions, stab marks, or burns.

— Document old traumatic lesions. Identify all healing versions of scars and hypopigmented or hyperpigmented marks.

1.   Record past trauma.

2.   The presence of old lesions can help identify perpetrators, indicate multiple abusers or a single abuser with repeated access to the child, or show lack of diligence of other adults.

— Bruise dating charts are based on color.

1.   Current knowledge does not support exact dating.

2.   Yellow coloration reliably indicates a passage of 18 to 24 hours since injury.[31,32]

3.   Beyond this, rely on personal experience, considering skin tone, depth and volume of bruising, and appearance of individual bruises.

— Distinguish lacerations from incisions.

1.   Lacerations are more common. Skin tears from blunt impact or stretching; nerves, blood vessels, and bands of connective tissue cross lacerations, creating bridges and irregular bases.

2.   Incisions appear as clean divisions of tissue and signify cutting with sharp objects.

— Inspect the nature, color, shape, size, and location of each lesion.

— Diagram lesions on a body drawing and photograph.

1.   Keep the plane of the film parallel to the plane of the injury.

2.   Use a size standard for comparison.

— Bruising:

1.   Any bruising on young infants is significant.[21]

2.   As children age, however, accidental bruising is more common, especially on anterior surfaces over bony prominences.

3.   The scalp, forehead, and shins are common bruise locations in children younger than 1 year.

— Examine marks for shape or pattern.

1.   Accidental injuries are typically ovate.[33]

2.   Patterns suggest specific forms of trauma.

3.   Clear bite marks may identify perpetrators.

4.   Grip marks, though uncommon, are associated with AHT.

   A. They comprise 2 to 5 ovate bruises in the shape of tips of a gripping hand.

   B. They are occasionally seen on the chest or upper arms, where the child may be held when shaken violently.

Abdomen

— Closely inspect, auscultate, and palpate the abdomen.

— Abuse-related injuries include liver contusions and lacerations, pancreatic injuries leading to pancreatitis and sometimes pseudocysts, and proximal small-bowel contusions and lacerations.[34-36]

— A compromised neurological state can make an examination unreliable. Some facilities image the abdomen of all children with compromised consciousness.

— Abdominal CT scans can detect complicating trauma.

Genitals

— Children hospitalized for abusive trauma typically are not victims of sexual abuse.[37]

— Use the frog-leg position and labial traction for female genitalia and supine knee-chest position for anal injuries.

— Use an otoscope for a well-illuminated and magnified view.

— With concerning findings, use a colposcope.

— If the child can tolerate it, conduct a prone knee-chest examination.

ADDITIONAL STUDIES
Cranial Imaging
— Most children have had head CT scans by the time AHT is suspected.

— CT scan is the preferred imaging technique because of its speed, ability to accommodate resuscitative equipment, and sensitivity to acute bleeding.

— Even when additional CT and magnetic resonance imaging (MRI) scans are not clinically necessary, they are desirable.

— Magnetic resonance imaging (MRI) is best for distinguishing chronic subdural from subarachnoid collections, detecting subacute and chronic subdural blood, and defining the nature and extent of parenchymal brain injuries.

— Acute SDHs, especially in the interhemispheric fissure; coexistence of acute and chronic SDHs; SDHs unaccompanied by skull fractures; and old brain injuries accompanying acute intracranial trauma are more common in abused infants.[9,12-14,37-40]

— See Chapter 3, Neuroradiology, for imaging details.

Skeletal Imaging
See Chapter 3, Neuroradiology.

Ophthalmology Examination
See Chapter 5, Ophthalmology.

Visceral Imaging
— Abdominal CT scans are useful in all unresponsive trauma victims and children with unexplained collapse.

— Internal injuries can be found when no outward signs of injury are visible.

— Injuries may only become visible on repeated scans, so all children with acute AHT should be followed for clinical and laboratory evidence of visceral injuries.

LABORATORY TESTING

— Laboratory data may be the first indication of AHT, show complications of head trauma, or reveal underlying conditions mistaken for abuse.

— Do not do a spinal tap in cases of known traumatic head injury. Avoid misdiagnosing mild or occult injuries as sepsis or meningitis, leading to the procedure.

— Do not assume bloody cerebrospinal fluid (CSF) indicates a traumatic tap; it may indicate an SAH from trauma.[41]

1. A similar cell count on the first and last tube indicates the blood is from CSF.

2. Finding cremated cells indicates they are from the CSF.

3. If bloody CSF is centrifuged and the supernate is xanthochromic, 2 to 4 hours may have passed since the initial trauma.[42]

— Blood tests should include at least electrolytes and a complete blood count including prothrombin time (PT), international normalized ratio (INR), partial thromboplastin time (PTT), aspartate aminotransferase (AST), alanine aminotransferase (ALT), and amylase.

— Complete blood count can indicate anemia in children with AHT.[27]

1. Anemia may be incidental, the result of earlier neglect, or the result of trauma.

2. A rapidly dropping hematocrit may indicate ongoing blood loss.

3. Anemia disproportionate to identifiable blood loss results from intravascular hemolysis from disseminated intravascular coagulation (DIC).

4. Assess white blood cell count for evidence of infection or leukemia.

5. Evaluate platelet count for thrombocytopenia.

6.   Evaluate PT, INR, and PTT to detect severe coagulation disorders causing bleeding in the head and eyes.

7.   It is necessary to definitively diagnose these disorders to treat and differentiate them from coagulation disorders caused by head trauma.

— Coagulopathy after head trauma is usually caused by DIC and predicts poor outcome.[43-46]

— AST, ALT, and amylase levels are sensitive indicators of occult internal injuries[47,48]; early in assessment, these levels may help detect hepatic or pancreatic injury not found radiographically.

— Hyponatremia is a delayed complication of head trauma and can lead to deterioration.

DIFFERENTIAL DIAGNOSIS
— When only intracranial bleeding or retinal hemorrhages are present, consider:

1.   Arteriovenous malformations

2.   Aneurysms

3.   Various metabolic disorders

4.   Coagulopathy (including late-onset hemorrhagic disease of the newborn)

5.   Leukemia

6.   Sickle cell anemia

— Avoid overdiagnosing these disorders; they are much less common than child abuse.

NATURE AND SEVERITY OF ABUSIVE TRAUMA
— The degree and nature of the trauma aid in identifying injuries as abusive.

— AHT is caused by unwarranted and unmistakable violence.

— Violent acceleration of the head causes extensive convexity and perifalcine SDHs.

1. The acceleration required varies with whether it is linear or rotational, lateral or sagittal, and impulse or impact initiated.

2. Peak acceleration, duration of acceleration, and total change in velocity must be considered.

— Some intracranial pathological conditions occur with small central retinal hemorrhages.

— Extensive, multilayered hemorrhages extending to the periphery are more specific for AHT and are produced by vitreoretinal traction during severe acceleration of the eye.

ACCIDENTAL TRAUMA

— Mild household trauma can cause skull fractures.

— Relatively mild trauma can produce EDHs and significant injuries.

1. Falls severe enough to cause skull fractures are also severe enough to cause EDHs, even when skull fractures do not occur.

2. EDHs are not specific to abuse and generally result from modest trauma and unfortunate chance.[49]

— Accidental head trauma can cause small SDHs and retinal hemorrhages.[50]

COMPLICATING VARIABLES

— Preexisting head injuries, including SDHs

1. Capillary-rich "neomembranes" at the margins of healing SDHs can rebleed spontaneously or after accidental injury.

2. Capillary rebleeding into chronic SDHs releases small amounts of blood, so the subdural collection grows slowly over time.

3. Sudden-onset symptoms may lead to the discovery of acute and chronic SDHs and the false impression of acute abusive injury.

4. When neurological deterioration occurs with rebleeding, evaluate for a mass effect. If images do not support a mass effect, the neurological change was caused by trauma.[51]

— Large CSF spaces surrounding the brain (*benign external hydrocephalus* or *expanded extra-axial space*)

1.   May be an isolated finding or accompanied by a large head circumference.

2.   Theoretically, normal vessels transversing the subarachnoid space from the dura mater to the brain are stretched so that the brain is freer to move in space; therefore, a child is vulnerable to injury caused by common household trauma. This concept is still being debated.[51]

3.   This theory does not explain situations involving SDHs with skull fractures, other skeletal injuries, direct brain parenchymal injuries, or classic retinal hemorrhages.

— The outcomes of abusive head injuries are significantly worse than the outcomes of accidental injuries.[12]

— Other factors:

1.   Time from injury to treatment

2.   Apnea

3.   Circulatory shock

4.   Coexisting abdominal injuries

5.   Evidence of strangulation

DEFINING THE MOMENT OF INJURY

RADIOLOGICAL EVIDENCE

— Skeletal injuries are dated based on the state of healing; intracranial injuries are dated by the appearance of subdural blood on CT scan and MRI.

— Only broad time ranges can be determined (eg, 7 to 14 days for periosteal elevation surrounding fractures and fewer than 7 days for hyperdense blood on CT scan).

— The timing is unclear with collections having a dark appearance.[52,53]

PATHOLOGICAL EVIDENCE

— Is obtained when children die or undergo surgery.

— Note organization of blood clots, formation of membranes around clots, and thickness of membranes in cell layers to determine the age of subdural hemorrhages.

— Only broad time ranges can be determined, but combining pathological and radiological data may clarify.

— If diffuse traumatic axonal injuries are documented on a pathological brain examination, timing based on symptom onset is more certain; however, axonal injuries have been found in nontraumatic injuries with the use of immunohistochemical staining techniques.[54,55]

— If the distribution and severity of axonal injury and neuropathological findings lead to a diagnosis of diffuse traumatic axonal injury, the patient must have lost consciousness for an extended period of time after the trauma and remained severely symptomatic until death.

LABORATORY EVIDENCE

— Is rarely helpful in determining the timing of injuries.

— If a lumbar puncture is performed, it may yield bloody CSF from an SAH.[41]

1. The blood is sometimes dismissed as the product of a traumatic tap.

2. If a xanthochromic supernate is found when bloody CSF is centrifuged, the blood is subarachnoid and SAH occurred several hours previously.[42]

3. This may document a delay in seeking care or help to identify the possible abuser.

SYMPTOMATIC EVIDENCE

— Is the most frequent evidence used to time traumatic events.

— Symptom onset begins at the time of trauma.[56-59]

— When a caregiver reports a sudden onset of dramatic and persistent symptoms in a child previously alert and well, that moment is presumed to be the moment of trauma.

— Mild symptoms can be recognized only after time passes.

— For symptom onset to be used effectively to time traumatic events, the condition of the child must be carefully assessed from the last clearly normal period.

— *Talk and die or deteriorate (TADD) syndrome:*

1. TADD is the concept that injured children can be conscious and relatively symptom-free for a time before deteriorating into a coma and/or dying. The *lucid interval* is defined as the time when a child has no symptoms observed by the caretaker. During this period, the child is often transferred to an innocent party before later developing severe symptoms, creating the impression that the innocent party hurt the child.

2. TADD is well-known in adults and can occur in children with head trauma[60-62] but is usually seen only with significant early symptoms after accidental trauma.

3. The cause is usually a growing intracranial mass compressing the brain.

4. Children are more likely to deteriorate from late-occurring diffuse brain swelling,[63-65] which can be caused by hyponatremia.[61,66,67]

5. An abused child can have an SDH, cerebral edema, normal electrolyte values, and be conscious and breathing when examined but later require ventilatory support and ultimately have permanent brain damage. This could be considered a lucid interval.

6. A child who is conscious and normal after head trauma may have an SDH but is highly unlikely to develop symptoms.[68]

7. Lucid intervals are reasonable in children with mild brain injury who deteriorate with late posttraumatic seizures, expanding intracranial mass, or hyponatremia.

OUTCOMES

— The outcomes of AHT are generally poor.

1. Death occurs in 10% to 25% of cases.

2. Moderate disability (eg, hemiparesis, borderline cognitive scores, more than one ongoing rehabilitative service, or placement in a

self-contained classroom) occurs in 65% of cases.

3.   Severe disability (eg, severe motor disability, severe cognitive impairment, or total dependence for daily care inappropriate for chronological age) occurs in 15% of cases.

— Even the minority who survive without serious disability may have long-term cognitive and behavioral effects.

— For children with accidental injuries, 55% have good recovery.

— Disability is greatest in patients who have definable parenchymal brain injuries.

REFERENCES

1.   Helfer ME, Kempe RS, Krugman RD. *The Battered Child*. Chicago, Ill: University of Chicago Press; 1997.

2.   US Dept of Health & Human Services, Administration on Children, Youth and Families. *Child Maltreatment 2000*. Washington, DC: US Government Printing Office; 2002. Available at: http://www.acf.hhs.gov/programs/cb/pubs/cm00/index.htm. Accessed April 13, 2005.

3.   DiScala C, Sege R, Li G, Reece RM. Child abuse and unintentional injuires: a 10-year retrospective. *Arch Pediatr Adolesc Med*. 2000;154:16-22.

4.   Reece RM, Sege R. Childhood head injuries: accidental or inflicted? *Arch Pediatr Adolesc Med*. 2000;154:11-15.

5.   Williams RA. Injuries in infants and small children resulting from witnessed and corroborated free falls. *J Trauma*. 1991;31:1350-1352.

6.   Selbst SM, Baker MD, Shames M. Bunk bed injuries. *Am J Dis Child*. 1990;144:721-723.

7.   Phelan KJ, Khoury J, Kalkwarf HJ, Lanphear BP. Trends and patterns of playground injuries in United States children and adolescents. *Ambul Pediatr*. 2001;1:227-233.

8. Luerssen TG, Bruce DA, Humphreys RP. Position statement on identifying the infant with nonaccidental central nervous system injury (the whiplash-shake syndrome). The American Society of Pediatric Neurosurgeons. *Pediatr Neurosurg.* 1993;19:170.

9. Jayawant S, Rawlinson A, Gibbon F, et al. Subdural haemorrhages in infants: population based study. *BMJ.* 1998;317:1558-1561.

10. Caffey J. Multiple fractures in the long bones of infants suffering from chronic subdural hematoma. *AJR Am J Roentgenol.* 1946;56: 163-173.

11. Kempe CH, Silverman FN, Steele B, Droegemueller W, Silver HK. The battered-child syndrome. *JAMA.* 1962;181:17-24.

12. Ewing-Cobbs L, Kramer L, Prasad M, et al. Neuroimaging, physical, and developmental findings after inflicted and noninflicted traumatic brain injury in young children. *Pediatrics.* 1998;102: 300-307.

13. Alexander R, Crabbe L, Sato Y, Smith W, Bennett T. Serial abuse in children who are shaken. *Am J Dis Child.* 1990;144:58-60.

14. Hymel KP, Rumack CM, Hay TC, Strain JD, Jenny C. Comparison of intracranial computed tomographic (CT) findings in pediatric abusive and accidental head trauma. *Pediatr Radiol.* 1997;27:743-747.

15. Chiaviello CT, Christoph RA, Bond GR. Stairway-related injuries in children. *Pediatrics.* 1994;94:679-681.

16. Joffe M, Ludwig S. Stairway injuries in children. *Pediatrics.* 1988; 82(pt 2):457-461.

17. Selbst SM, Baker MD, Shames M. Bunk bed injuries. *Am J Dis Child.* 1990;144:721-723.

18. Gurdjian ES, Webster JE, Lissner HR. The mechanism of skull fracture. *Radiology.* 1950;54:313-339.

19. Hobbs CJ. Skull fracture and the diagnosis of abuse. *Arch Dis Child.* 1984;59:246-252.

20. Wheeler DS, Shope TR. Depressed skull fracture in a 7-month-old who fell from bed. *Pediatrics*. 1997;100:1033-1034.

21. Sugar NF, Taylor JA, Feldman KW. Bruises in infants and toddlers: those who don't cruise rarely bruise. Puget Sound Pediatric Research Network. *Arch Pediatr Adolesc Med*. 1999;153:399-403.

22. Wahl NG, Woodall BN. Hypothermia in shaken infant syndrome. *Pediatr Emerg Care*. 1995;11:233-234.

23. Woelfle J, Kreft B, Emons D, Haverkamp F. Subdural hemorrhage as an initial sign of glutaric aciduria type 1: a diagnostic pitfall. *Pediatr Radiol*. 1996;26:779-781.

24. Kleinman PK, Spevak MR. Soft tissue swelling and acute skull fracture. *J Pediatr*. 1992;121(pt 1):737-739.

25. Feldman KW. Patterned abusive bruises of the buttocks and the pinna. *Pediatrics*. 1992;90:633-636.

26. Kivlin JD, Simons KB, Lazoritz S, Ruttum MS. Shaken baby syndrome. *Ophthalmology*. 2000;107:1246-1254.

27. Hadley MH, Sontag VK, Rekate HL, Murphy A. The infant whiplash-shake injury syndrome: a clinical and pathological study. *Neurosurgery*. 1989;24:536-540.

28. Feldman KW, Weinberger E, Milstein JM, Fligner CL. Cervical spine MRI in abused infants. *Child Abuse Negl*. 1997;21:199-205.

29. Gleckner AM, Kessler SC, Smith TW. Periadventitial extracranial vertebral artery hemorrhage in a case of shaken baby syndrome. *J Forensic Sci*. 2000;45:1151-1153.

30. Saternus KS, Kernback-Wighton G, Oehmichen M. The shaking trauma in infants–kinetic chains. *Forensic Sci Int*. 2000;109:203-213.

31. Langlois NE, Greshan GA. The ageing of bruises: a review and study of the colour changes with time. *Forensic Sci Int*. 1991;50:227-238.

32. Stephenson T, Bialas Y. Estimation of the age of bruising. *Arch Dis Child*. 1996;74:53-55.

33. Carpenter RF. The prevalence and distribution of bruising in babies. *Arch Dis Child*. 1999;30:363-366.

34. Ledbetter DJ, Harch EI Jr, Feldman KW, Fligner CL, Tapper D. Diagnostic and surgical implications of child abuse. *Arch Surg*. 1988;123:1101-1105.

35. Ng CS, Hall CM, Shaw DG. The range of visceral manifestations of non-accidental injury. *Arch Dis Child*. 1997;77:167-174.

36. Sivit CJ, Taylor GA, Eichelberger MR. Visceral injury in battered children: a changing perspective. *Radiology*. 1989;173:659-661.

37. Reece RM, Sege R. Childhood head injuries: accidental or inflicted? *Arch Pediatr Adolesc Med*. 2000;154:11-15.

38. Ewing-Cobbs L, Prasad M, Kramer L, et al. Acute neuroradiologic findings in young children with inflicted or noninflicted traumatic brain injury. *Childs Nerv Syst*. 2000;16:25-34.

39. Goldstein B, Kelly MM, Bruton D, Cox C. Inflicted versus accidental head injury in critically injured children. *Crit Care Med*. 1993;21:1328-1332.

40. Wells RG, Vetter C, Laud R. Intracrantial hemorrhage in children younger than 3 years: prediction of intent. *Arch Pediatr Adolesc Med*. 2002;156:252-257.

41. Spear RM, Chadwick D, Peterson BM. Fatalities associated with misinterpretation of bloody cerebrospinal fluid in "shaken baby syndrome." *Am J Dis Child*. 1992;146:1415-1417.

42. Greenfield JG, Carmichael FA. *Cerebrospinal Fluid in Clinical Diagnosis*. London, England: McMillan; 1925.

43. Hymel KP, Abshire TC, Lukey DW, Jenny C. Coagulopathy in pediatric abusive head trauma. *Pediatrics*. 1997;99:371-375.

44. Becker S, Schneider W, Kreuz W, Jacobi G, Scharrer I, Nowak-Gottl U. Posttrauma coagulation and fibrinolysis in children suffering from severe cerebrocranial trauma. *Eur J Pediatr*. 1999; 158(suppl):197-203.

45. Chiaretti A, Pezzotti P, Mestrovic J, et al. The influence of hemo-coagulative disorders on the outcome of children with head injury. *Pediatr Neurosurg.* 2001;34:131-137.

46. Vavilala MS, Dunbar PJ, Rivara FP, Lam AM. Coagulopathy predicts poor outcome following head injury in children less than 16 years of age. *J Neurosurg Anesthesiol.* 2001;13:13-18.

47. Coant PN, Kornberg AE, Brody AS, Edwards-Holmes K. Markers for occult liver injury in cases of physical abuse in children. *Pediatrics.* 1992;89:274-278.

48. Holmes JF, Sokolove PE, Land C, Kuppermann N. Identification of intraabdominal injuries in children hospitalized following blunt torso trauma. *Acad Emerg Med.* 1999;6:799-806.

49. Shugerman RP, Paez A, Grossman DC, Feldman KW, Grady MS. Epidural hemorrhage: is it abuse? *Pediatrics.* 1996;97:664-668.

50. Duhaime AC, Christian C, Armonda R, Hunter J, Hertle R. Disappearing subdural hematomas in children. *Pediatr Neurosurg.* 1996;25:116-122.

51. Hymel KP, Jenny C, Block RW. Intracranial hemorrhage and re-bleeding in suspected victims of abusive head trauma: addressing forensic controversies. *Child Maltreat.* 2002;7:329-348.

52. Dias MS, Backstrom J, Falk M, Li V. Serial radiography in the infant shaken impact syndrome. *Pediatr Neurosurg.* 1998;29:77-85.

53. Vinchon M, Noizet O, Defoort-Dhellemmes S, Soto-Ares G, Dhellemmes P. Infantile subdural hematomas due to traffic accidents. *Pediatr Neurosurg.* 2002;37:245-253.

54. Geddes JF, Whitwell HL, Graham DI. Traumatic axonal injury: practical issues for diagnosis in medicolegal cases. *Neuropathol Appl Neurobiol.* 2000;26:105-116.

55. Shannon P, Smith CR, Deck J, Ang LC, Ho M, Becher L. Axonal injury and the neuropathology of shaken baby syndrome. *Acta Neuropathol (Berl).* 1998;95:625-631.

56. Duhaime AC, Christian CW, Rorke LB, Zimmerman RA. Nonaccidental head injury in infants—the "shaken-baby syndrome." *N Engl J Med*. 1998;339:1822-1829.

57. Starling SP, Patel S, Burke BL, Sirotnak AP, Stronks S, Rosquist P. Analysis of perpetrator admissions to inflicted traumatic brain injury in children. *Arch Pediatr Adolesc Med*. 2004;158:454-458.

58. Starling SP, Holden JR, Jenny C. Abusive head trauma: the relationship of perpetrators to their victims. *Pediatrics*. 1995;95:259-262.

59. Gilles EE, Nelson MD Jr. Cerebral complications of nonaccidental head injury in childhood. *Pediatr Neurol*. 1998;19:119-128.

60. Hendrick EB, Harwood-Hash DC, Hudson AR. Head injuries in children, a survey of 4465 consecutive cases at the hospital for sick children, Toronto, Canada. *Clin Neurosurg*. 1964;11:46-65.

61. Humphreys RP, Hendrick EB, Hoffman MJ. The head-injured child who "talks and dies." A report of 4 cases. *Childs Nerv Syst*. 1990;6:139-142.

62. Snoek JW, Minderhoud JM, Wilmink JT. Delayed deterioration following mild head injury in children. *Brain*. 1984;107(pt 1):15-36.

63. Aldrich EF, Eisenberg HM, Saydjari C, et al. Diffuse brain swelling in severely head-injured children. A report from the NIH Traumatic Coma Data Bank. *Neurosurgery*. 1992;76:450-454.

64. Bruce DA, Alvi A, Bilaniuk L, Dolinskas C, Obrist W, Uzzell B. Diffuse cerebral swelling following head injuries in children: the syndrome of "malignant brain edema." *J Neurosurg*. 1981;54:170-178.

65. Lobato RD, Rivas JJ, Gomez PA, et al. Head injured patients who talk and deteriorate into coma. Analysis of 211 cases studied with computerized tomography. *J Neurosurg*. 1991;75:256-261.

66. Vingerhoets F, de Tribolet N. Hyponatremia hypo-osmolarity in neurosurgical patients. "Appropriate secretion of ADH" and "cerebral salt wasting syndrome." *Acta Neurochir (Wien)*. 1988;91:50-54.

67. Zafonte RD, Mann NR. Cerebral salt wasting syndrome in brain injury patients: a potential cause of hyponatremia. *Arch Phys Med Rehabil.* 1997;78:540-542.

68. Greenes DS, Schutzman SA. Clinical indicators of intracranial injury in head-injured infants. *Pediatrics.* 1999;104(pt 1):861-867.

Chapter 2

BIOMECHANICS

Betty Spivack, MD

BASIC MECHANICS

PHYSICS OF LINEAR MOTION

— The principle of *inertia*, or resistance to change of linear motion, is that objects continue in a linear motion with constant velocity, measured in meters per second, unless a force is applied to alter that motion.

— *Mass* (m) is measured in kilograms. It is a measure of the resistance to change in motion.

— *Force* (f) is measured in newtons. It is the energy needed to change linear velocity, and it is proportional to both mass and acceleration.

— *Acceleration* (a) is measured in meters per second. It is the change in velocity per unit time.

1. The relationship is expressed as:

$$F = ma$$

2. After a force is applied, the linear velocity of objects changes because of acceleration produced by force.

3. The relationship between acceleration, duration of acceleration (t), original velocity (v_0), terminal velocity (v_t), and distance traveled (d) is as follows:

$$v_t = v_0 + at$$

$$d = \tfrac{1}{2}\,at^2$$

— *Work* (W) is measured in joules or newton-meters. It is the result of force applied through a distance.

— *Energy* (E) is measured in joules. It is the capacity to do work.

1. For a given injury to occur, sufficient energy must be available to do the needed work on the body.

2. Energy can arise from motion (kinetic energy) or position (potential energy).

3. Potential energy represents the effect of acceleration caused by gravity should the object fall from a height (h).

4. Acceleration resulting from gravity (g) is 9.8 m/s^2.

— The principle of *conservation of energy* is that the total energy of a system (kinetic plus potential) remains constant throughout object movements and interactions within the system. The following equations govern these parameters:

$$\textbf{W = Fd}$$
$$\mathbf{E_{(kinetic)} = \tfrac{1}{2}\, mv^2}$$
$$\mathbf{E_{(potential)} = mgh}$$

— A falling object initially at rest has all its potential energy converted into kinetic energy, except what is lost to friction from air resistance.

1. Air resistance has little effect on the human body at heights less than 10 to 15 m and only small effect at heights less than 50 m.

2. As the height from which a person's fall increases, air resistance increases. A freely falling body cannot reach a terminal velocity greater than 67 m/s (150 mph).

3. The following equations explain the relationships between height, falling time, and terminal velocities in objects falling from rest at lower heights:

$$\mathbf{t = \sqrt{(2h/g)}} \quad \textbf{(if starting from rest)}$$
$$\mathbf{vt = \sqrt{(2gh)}}$$

PHYSICS OF ANGULAR MOTION
— Force continually applied to an object in linear motion, in a direction perpendicular to the linear motion, causes the object to move in a circle around the source of the force.

— The force needed to change rotational velocity (ω), measured in radians per second, of an object depends on inertia or mass and on distribution of mass relative to the axis of rotation.

— Resistance to change in rotational motion = moment of inertia (I) and is governed by the following equation:

$$I = \int L2 \; dm \; \text{or} \; \sum mL2$$

— If the object is a point mass or very small and far away from the axis of rotation, the moment of inertia is effectively mL2, where L is the radius of rotation.

— If the object is a cylinder, sphere, box, or irregular form rotating around its own center of gravity, the calculation varies.

— ***Rotational acceleration*** (α) is measured in radians per second squared. It is a change in rotational velocity per unit time.

1. It requires force be applied perpendicular to the linear motion of the object.

2. The rotational effect of the force is called ***torque.***

— During rotation, angular momentum is maintained.

1. Angular momentum is the product of the moment of inertia and angular velocity.

2. If the moment of inertia increases, angular velocity decreases.

3. If the moment of inertia declines, angular velocity increases.

RESPONSE TO LOADING FORCES

— If a force or load is applied to an object, the effect on the object depends on factors such as size of the load, direction of application, rate at which the force is applied, surface area over which it is applied, and material properties of the object.

— When force is applied, it is distributed evenly over the surface area of application, causing stress (σ), which is measured in pascals (equivalent to newtons per meter squared).

— The ***ultimate strength*** of an object is the maximum stress it can tolerate before mechanical failure or rupture.

— When 2 objects interact, they exert equivalent forces on each other. If the exerted stress exceeds the ultimate strength of 1 object, that object breaks.

— The limiting factor of ultimate strength is that more direct damage occurs when the force is concentrated in a small area than when it is diffused over a larger area.

Elastic Deformation
— Objects may deform elastically without rupture (**Figure 2-1**).[1]

— Elastic deformation is proportional to the force applied and is reversible. When the force is removed, the object returns to its original state.

— The proportional change in dimension is called ***strain***, which is a nondimensional measurement. When an object exceeds its maximum strain, it ruptures.

— The elastic modulus (E, Young's modulus, or modulus of rigidity) is the ratio of stress to strain and is a constant for any uniform material.

— Very elastic substances (eg, rubber) have a large strain with a relatively low stress; their elastic modulus is small.

— Rigid substances (eg, concrete) have very little deformation even with large forces and have a large elastic modulus.

— Elastic deformation stores energy, which is released when the substance returns to its initial state and can be used to perform work.

— Viscoelastic substances have elastic properties that vary depending on the application rate of a load (**Figures 2-2-a** and **b**). Such substances are stiff when a force is applied rapidly but more elastic

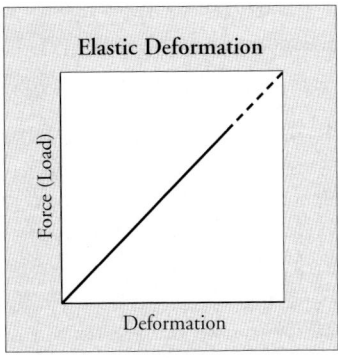

Figure 2-1. *In an elastic deformation, the degree of temporary deformation is directly proportional to the applied force.*[1]

when the loading rate is decreased.

— For events of short duration, strain is proportional to force X time.

1. Because F = ma and v = at, this time dependence of response implies that, for viscoelastic substances, velocity rather than acceleration is a critical threshold for short-term events.

2. Events that last longer are more influenced by acceleration.

— In general, biological materials behave elastically until stress exceeds a *yield point.* After this the material deforms nonelastically (not proportionally to the force exerted).

1. This can be associated with *plastic deformation,* which is a permanent deformation without true rupture. Energy used for plastic deformation is not recoverable.

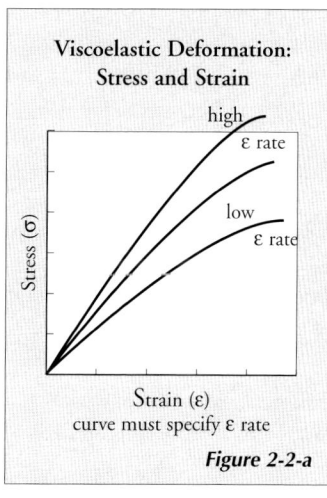

**Viscoelastic Deformation:
Stress and Strain**

high

ε rate

low

ε rate

Stress (σ)

Strain (ε)

curve must specify ε rate

Figure 2-2-a

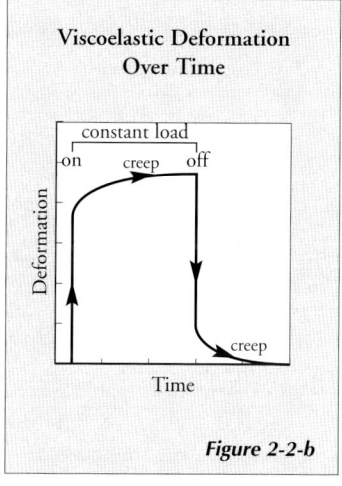

**Viscoelastic Deformation
Over Time**

constant load

on   creep   off

Deformation

creep

Time

Figure 2-2-b

Figure 2-2-a. *Viscoelastic substances are relatively rigid when forces are rapidly applied. Low strain rates lead to greater deformation with less stress.*[1]

Figure 2-2-b. *Viscoelastic substances develop a rapid, elastic response to applied loads, but then experience a slow, continuing deformation or "creep" until the load is discontinued. The elastic deformation is rapidly reversible, the creep may slowly dissipate after cessation of the load.*[1]

2. With continued force application, stress increases until the ultimate strength of the material is reached and rupture occurs. Energy released in rupture is not recoverable.

3. Most biological materials are viscoelastic and behave differently under conditions of dynamic and static loading. During dynamic loading, response depends on rate of loading.

— An object's response to loading is also sensitive to effects of scale.

1. If objects are increased in size proportionally, volume, mass, and weight increase as a function of the cube of the linear dimension. However, surface area increases as a function of the square of linear dimension.

2. As a result, the stress derived from supporting the object's own weight increases, raising the chance that the stress will exceed the yield point or ultimate strength.

— The result of an impact event depends on several factors.

1. As the surface area of contact increases, stress generated by the impact decreases, reducing the chance that the stress will exceed the yield point or ultimate strength.

2. Elastic properties of both impacting materials determine the degree of deformation.

3. The sum of deformations determines the distance traveled during deceleration and therefore also the interval over which velocity decreases to zero.

4. The more deformable the 2 substances, the longer the impact event is and the lower the deceleration, force of impact, and generated stress of impact are.

5. The greater the elasticity of a substance, the more likely it is to bounce after impact.

6. The energy used for bouncing is not available to cause permanent injury.

7. Viscoelastic properties of impacting substances determine the

extent to which impact times affect the nature and degree of resulting injury.

BIOMECHANICAL BASIS OF TRAUMATIC BRAIN INJURY

— Following are crucial material properties of cerebral tissue[2]:

1. The brain is roughly uniform in density. Although there are small differences in density, nerve tissue, blood, and cerebrospinal fluid (CSF) all approximate the density of water.

2. The brain is very resistant to compressive strain.

3. The brain is not rigid. It changes shape easily with small applications of local force.

4. The rigidity of the skull is much greater than the rigidity of the brain.

5. The shapes of the skull and the brain are important in determining the location of injuries.

HOLBOURN'S MODEL

— The brain behaves like other biological tissues, with injuries arising mainly from shear strains rather than tensile or compressive strains. Therefore skull distortion causes maximal shearing close to the site of impact.

1. Waves of compression and tension after impact and skull distortion cause comparatively little injury.

2. Diffuse injuries, including concussions and contrecoup injuries, usually result from acceleration effects, especially rotational acceleration, causing the most shearing.

3. Linear acceleration causes compressive loads with little shear strain and is not a major force in injury.

— Effects of brain viscoelasticity:

1. In short-duration events, rotational velocity is the critical threshold for injury.

2. In long-duration events, rotational acceleration is more important.

3. The transition between these 2 types of events occurs at an interval between 2 and 200 milliseconds (msec).

4. Static loads associated with minimal head acceleration (eg, crush injuries) are unlikely to be associated with concussions.

— The model in **Figure 2-3** corroborates Holbourn's concept of rotational injury as the source of contrecoup contusions and shows where potential bridging vein rupture results from rotation.

— Sagittal rotation from occipital impact causes maximal superficial shear along the midline, with significant frontal contusion and relatively little injury in the cerebellar area.

— The model is limited by the lack of separating membranes and failure to reflect the differences in density of the cortex, white matter, and CSF.

OTHER STUDY MODEL FINDINGS

— In short-duration events, as the interval of acceleration decreases, the threshold of rotational acceleration increases in inverse proportion.

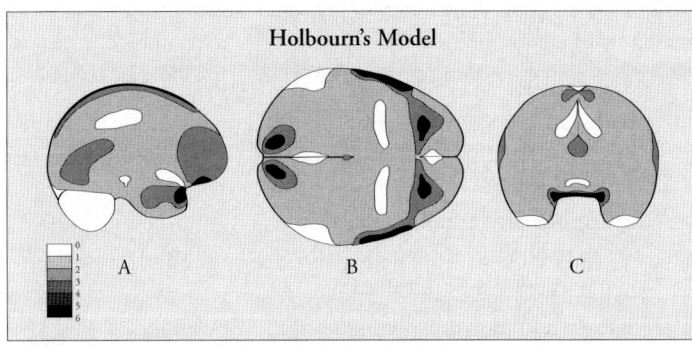

Figure 2-3. Holbourn's model. Distribution of shearing injuries in gelatin model of brain subjected to rotational forces in varying axes. Degree of injury increases with darkness of diagram. Sagittal rotation following blow to occiput (A). Horizontal rotation following blow to jaw (B). Coronal rotation following blow to ear (C). Adapted from Holbourn,[2] from The Lancet with permission from Elsevier.

— The most common injuries in short duration events are small para-sagittal subdural hematomas, often associated with superficial para-sagittal frontoparietal contusions.

— Animals that do not lose consciousness generally do not have macroscopic injuries.

— Critical thresholds for rotational velocity and acceleration are about 50% higher when head motion is not associated with impact.[3,4]

— The natural frequency of wave transmission in the brain ranges from 5 to 10 Hz in animals studied and is anticipated to be 4 to 5 Hz in humans.[3,5]

1. The range of natural frequency is critical in determining transition points between long- and short-duration events and predicted acceleration thresholds.

2. Higher natural frequencies lead to higher rotational acceleration thresholds and a quicker transition to long-duration events.

— Purely translational accelerations do not produce concussions even though concussions are easily elicited by comparable or smaller tangential accelerations with rotational head motion.[6,7]

— Acute subdural hematomas (ASDH) are most likely with relatively high strain rates and short acceleration or deceleration intervals.[8,9]

— As pulse duration increases above 5 msec, apparent rotational acceleration thresholds also increase. Diffuse axonal injuries (DAI) and prolonged traumatic comas occur with pulse durations greater than 6 msec and oblique or coronal rotation.[8,9]

1. The separation of DAI and ASDH kinematic patterns is paralleled by the relative frequency of ASDH and rarity of DAI in falls and assaults (ie, injury mechanisms with brief acceleration or deceleration impulses).

2. In adults, DAI is more common and ASDH less common after motor vehicle crashes.

3. DAI and ASDH can coexist.[10]

— Mechanism of traumatic axonal injuries:

1. The principal site of damage is Ranvier's nodes[11] between successive segments of the myelin sheath.

2. In the first few hours after injury, organelle and axolemma damage develops at Ranvier's nodes.[11,12]

3. Subtle changes in organelles and axolemma are seen with metabolic changes in axons, causing excessive calcium ion accumulation in the axoplasm and other metabolic derangements.[11-15]

4. Severe altered metabolisms may cause axonal degeneration.

5. Initial shearing injuries appear time limited.

6. Associated organelle injuries cause secondary axonal damages from toxic metabolic environments.

7. Organelle damage, but not shearing damage, can occur from other mechanisms of secondary injury (eg, hypoxic-ischemic encephalopathy).

MODERN PARADIGM OF TRAUMATIC BRAIN INJURY

— Traumatic brain injuries are classified by mechanism of injury rather than site (**Table 2-1**).[14-17] This can be confusing clinically because some injuries are caused by more than one mechanism.

Table 2-1. Biomechanical Classification of Traumatic Brain Injuries		
CLASSIFICATION OF INJURY	DESCRIPTION	EXAMPLES
Primary Injuries	Direct result of mechanical forces acting on the external and intracranial tissues of the head	
Focal Injuries	Arise from contact forces and translational acceleration events	

(continued)

Table 2-1. *(continued)*

CLASSIFICATION OF INJURY	DESCRIPTION	EXAMPLES
Contact	Focal results of skull deformation; all require direct application of force to the head, but the impact interval can be brief or prolonged and quasistatic	Soft tissue injuries, skull fractures or deformations, epidural hematomas, subdural hematomas, superficial cortical contusions, lacerations
Translational inertia	Results from acceleration-deceleration events associated with a head that has been put in motion before, during, or after the trauma; rotational inertial forces are more injurious than translational inertial events	Cortical contusions (contrecoup), lacerations, intracerebral hematomas, subdural hematomas, subarachnoid hemorrhages, petechial hemorrhages
Diffuse Injuries	Associated with immediate alterations of consciousness, brief or prolonged; always associated with rotational inertial events with or without cranial impact	
Rotational inertia	Rotational forces are most likely to induce shearing injuries at interfaces between structures that differ in density or other material properties; injuries are highly correlated with immediate loss of consciousness and traumatic axonal injury	Concussions, subdural hematomas, subarachnoid hemorrhages, petechial hemorrhages, contusional tears, traumatic axonal injuries
Secondary Injuries	Result from complications caused by vascular and metabolic derangements arising from initial trauma	Neurological injuries
Hypoxic-ischemic injuries		Cerebral edemas (vasogenic, cytotoxic), infarctions, metabolic derangements
Pressure injuries		Infarctions, herniation syndromes

— Concussions, traumatic comas, and DAIs only occur with diffuse injuries.

— ASDHs can arise from contact events, translational inertial events, or rotational inertial events.

1. Contact-type ASDHs underlie sites of skull fractures or temporary skull deformations and are the result of focal ruptures of bridging veins or direct lacerations of venous sinuses by bone fragments from a fractured skull or penetrating foreign body.

2. Inertial ASDHs are more likely bilateral, parasagittal, and widely distributed. The size and site of hematomas do not reliably differentiate between contact and inertial ASDH.

   A. A contact hematoma from lacerated transverse sinus associated with depressed skull fracture may be extremely large because of large blood flow to the venous sinus and can extend into parasagittal spaces by proximity.

   B. Parasagittal or interhemispheric ASDH more typically arises from rotational inertial mechanisms associated with sagittal rotation and tearing of multiple bridging veins. These are often small but widely distributed parasagittally or over 1 or both cerebral hemispheres and are called skim or thin film SDHs.

— Differences in density and other material properties yield differing response times to change in motion, causing slippage at the interfaces.

1. This is most notable at the junction of gray and white matter.

2. Petechial hemorrhages are often seen in this zone after head trauma with a significant rotational component. More substantial gliding contusions (contusional tears) are also possible.

3. Such injuries highly correlate with immediate loss of consciousness and traumatic axonal injury.

— Factors promoting contact injuries include small surface area of contact, rigid impacting material, and fixation of the head (impedes movement arising from impact).

1. There is no immediate loss of consciousness with pure contact events unless the brainstem is involved in focal trauma.

2. Delayed loss of consciousness is seen with secondary injuries.

3. Mass effect from an epidural hematoma may cause pressure gradients, leading to uncal or central herniation. The herniation sequence causes loss of consciousness.

— Factors in inertial injuries include rotational motion of the head before impact, subsequent to impact, or unassociated with impact to the head; large area of impact; and relatively nonrigid impacting material.

1. The threshold injury in rotational inertia is concussion.

2. Pathologic findings (eg, ASDH) are not attributable to rotational events if the patient did not have a concussion.

3. Contact, translational, and rotational inertial injuries may coexist.

— Axons may degenerate secondarily from hypoxic-ischemic or neurotoxic complications. Traumatic axonal injuries must be distinguished from white matter injuries caused by other sources.

1. Not all traumatic axonal injuries are diffuse. The site of injury indicates the mechanism.[18]

2. Ommaya's ***centripetal theory of cerebral concussion*** suggests the severity sequence in axonal injuries.[17]

    A. Increasing severity of disturbances in level of consciousness is caused by mechanically induced strains at progressively deeper brain levels.

    B. The effects of the sequence always begin at brain surfaces in mild cases and extend inward to diencephalon and mesencephalon core in the most severe cases.

NOTE: The centripetal theory is currently an incompletely tested hypothesis.

— Conclusions:

1. In head injuries severe enough to cause traumatic comas (grade III concussive injuries and above), primary injuries are most severe in the cortical and subcortical structures with relative sparing of the

rostral brainstem. Brainstems recover well with grade III and some grade IV injuries.

2. Primary damage from inertial mechanisms does not occur with injuries in the rostral brainstem unless associated diffuse brain damage is present.

3. Confusion and memory disturbances can occur without loss of consciousness, but the reverse is not seen, except with delayed loss of consciousness caused by secondary phenomena.

BIOMECHANICS OF PEDIATRIC ABUSIVE HEAD TRAUMA

— Rotational acceleration-deceleration injuries, generated by shaking, determine the type and severity of abusive head trauma (AHT).

— Children who die suddenly or unexpectedly from abuse have small or skim subdural hematomas, typically parafalcine in location; retinal hemorrhages; seizures; apnea or bradycardia during examination; and poor outcome/high mortality.

— Diffuse axonal and white matter injuries occur in fatal cases.[19,20]

— Bruises and skull fractures are more common in fatal cases.

— Evidence of impact is not found until postmortem examination in many fatal cases.[21,22]

SHAKEN BABY SYNDROME/SHAKEN IMPACT SYNDROME

— Even soft impacts producing visible soft tissue injuries can markedly increase pathologic loads of the brain and surrounding tissues.

— Human infant white matter has significantly less myelin than adult white matter.

— Axonal injury is principally in the region of Ranvier's nodes, which has myelin sheath gaps.[11,12]

— Immature, undermyelinated axons are more susceptible to axonal injury than fully myelinated adult axons.[23]

— Undermyelinized infant brains are significantly more susceptible to rotational inertial injuries than fully myelinized adult brains.

— Immature brains are less susceptible to impact injuries than adult brains.

— Shaking produces repetitive oscillatory motion due to periodic reapplication of impulses and can lower thresholds for injury.

1. Repetitive loading may lead to subclinical microtrauma, causing increased susceptibility to injury from low levels of rotation.

2. Harmonic amplification of the energy, force, and stresses experienced by the brain may occur if the frequency of shaking is a low integer multiple of the natural frequency of the skull and intracranial contents. Thresholds for injury depend on the number of shakes and the characteristics of each individual shake. Threshold levels for inertial injuries are lower for the more shakes administered.

3. Both mechanisms may be relevant to shaking injuries.

— Many infants with inflicted head trauma have evidence of head impact. In fatal cases, even higher proportions are seen.[21,22,24]

— Milder degrees of injury show less likelihood of head impact.[25] Intracranial injuries are predominantly SDHs and retinal hemorrhages.

— There is a high incidence of apnea in infants with AHT.[26,27]

— The brains of infants who die of AHT often show hypoxic-ischemic encephalopathy.[18,28,29]

— High levels of inflammatory and toxic metabolites are found in pediatric traumatic brain injuries, but much higher levels are found in AHT.

— Many of these substances are directly neurotoxic, contributing to the dismal outcomes of children with AHT compared to survivors of accidental head trauma.[24,30,31]

— Retinal hemorrhages:

1. Correlate more strongly with AHT from shaking than accidental head trauma, even when accidental injuries are severe.[32-35]

2. Are occasionally incurred in household accidents[36] but consist of

few small unilateral hemorrhages isolated to the posterior pole. They are not caused by typical short falls.

3. Mechanisms of injury include orbital shaking and vitreous traction directly resulting from shaking. This helps explain the common finding of retinal hemorrhages extending to the far periphery of the retina, traumatic retinoschisis, optic nerve sheath hemorrhages, and axonal optic nerve injuries in infants with AHT.

4. Use of beta-amyloid precursor protein staining can identify traumatic axonal injuries of the optic nerve.[37]

5. Retinal injuries are rarely seen in children with traumatic brain injury from other mechanisms.

— Skeletal injuries:

1. Are frequently associated with AHT.

2. Rib fractures, especially of the posterior ribs, are the most frequently identified skeletal injury.

3. Fractures are produced by levering the paravertebral portion of the rib against the transverse process of the vertebrae when the chest is forcefully squeezed while the back is unsupported.[38,39]

4. This fracture pattern reflects the most common hand positions during shaking.

5. Rib fractures are not produced by cardiopulmonary resuscitation in infants.

REFERENCES

1. Cochran GVB. *A Primer of Orthopaedic Biomechanics*. New York, NY: Churchill Livingstone; 1982.

2. Holbourn AHS. Mechanics of head injuries. *Lancet*. 1943;2:438-441.

3. Ommaya AK, Fisch FJ, Mahone RM, Corrao P, Letcher F. Comparative tolerances for cerebral concussion by head impact and whiplash injury in primates. SAE; 1980. Reprinted in: Backaitis SH, ed. *Biomechanics of Impact Injury and Injury Tolerances of the*

Head Neck Complex. Warrendale, Pa: Society of Automotive Engineers; 1993:265-274.

4. Ommaya AK, Hirsch AE. Tolerances for cerebral concussion from head impact and whiplash in primates. *J Biomech.* 1971;4:13-21.

5. Ommaya AK, Grubb RL Jr, Naumann RA. Coup and contre-coup injury: observations on the mechanics of visible brain injuries in the rhesus monkey. *J Neurosurg.* 1971;35:503-516.

6. Gennarelli TA, Thibault LE, Ommaya AK. Pathophysiologic responses to rotational and translational accelerations of the head. SAE; 1972. Reprinted in: Backaitis SH, ed. *Biomechanics of Impact Injury and Injury Tolerances of the Head Neck Complex.* Warrendale, Pa: Society of Automotive Engineers; 1993:411-423.

7. Hirsch AE, Ommaya AK. Protection from brain injury: the relative significance of translational and rotational motions of the head after impact. SAE; 1970. Reprinted in: Backaitis SH, ed. *Biomechanics of Impact Injury and Injury Tolerances of the Head Neck Complex.* Warrendale, Pa: Society of Automotive Engineers; 1993: 275-282.

8. Gennarelli TA, Thibault LE, Adams JH, Graham DI, Thompson CJ, Marcincin RP. Diffuse axonal injury and traumatic coma in the primate. *Ann Neurol.* 1982;12:564-574.

9. Gennarelli TA, Thibault LE, Tomel G, Wiser R, Graham D, Adams J. Directional dependence of axonal brain injury due to centroidal and non-centroidal acceleration. SAE; 1987. Reprinted in: Backaitis SH, ed. *Biomechanics of Impact Injury and Injury Tolerances of the Head Neck Complex.* Warrendale, Pa: Society of Automotive Engineers; 1993:595-599.

10. Adams JH, Graham DI, Murray LS, Scott G. Diffuse axonal injury due to nonmissile head injury in humans: an analysis of 45 cases. *Ann Neurol.* 1982;12:557-563.

11. Maxwell WL, Watt C, Graham DI, Gennarelli TA. Ultrastructural evidence of axonal shearing as a result of lateral acceleration of the

head in non-human primates. *Acta Neuropathol (Berl)*. 1993; 86: 136-144.

12. Gennarelli TA, Tipperman R, Maxwell WL, Graham DI, Adams JH, Irvine A. Traumatic damage to the nodal axolemma: an early secondary injury. *Acta Neurochir Suppl (Wien)*. 1993;57:49-52.

13. Erb DE, Povlishock JT. Axonal damage in severe traumatic brain injury: an experimental study in cat. *Acta Neuropathol (Berl)*. 1988;76:347-358.

14. Gennarelli TA. Mechanisms of brain injury. *J Emerg Med*. 1993;11 (suppl 1):5-11.

15. McIntosh TK, Smith DH, Meaney DF, Kotapka M, Gennarelli TA, Graham DI. Neuropathological sequelae of traumatic brain injury: relationship to neurochemical and biomechanical mechanisms. *Lab Invest*. 1996;74:315-342.

16. Bandak FA. On the mechanics of impact neurotrauma: a review and critical synthesis. *J Neurotrauma*. 1995;11:635-649.

17. Ommaya AK. Head injury mechanisms and the concept of preventive management: a review and critical synthesis. *J Neurotrauma*. 1995;12:527-546.

18. Geddes JF, Vowles GH, Hackshaw AK, Nickols CD, Scott IS, Whitwell HL. Neuropathology of inflicted head injury in children. II. Microscopic brain injury in infants. *Brain*. 2001;124(pt 7):184-186.

19. Calder IM, Hill I, Scholtz CL. Primary brain trauma in non-accidental injury. *J Clin Pathol*. 1984;37:1095-1100.

20. Spevak MR, Kleinman PK, Belanger PL, Primack C, Richmond JM. Cardiopulmonary resuscitation and rib fractures in infants. A postmortem radiologic-pathologic study. *JAMA*. 1994;272:617-618.

21. Duhaime AC, Gennarelli TA, Thibault LE, Bruce DA, Margulies SS, Wiser R. The shaken baby syndrome. A clinical, pathological, and biomechanical study. *J Neurosurg*. 1987;66:409-415.

22. Hahn YS, Raimondi AJ, McLone DG, Yamanouchi Y. Traumatic mechanisms of head injury in child abuse. *Childs Brain*. 1983;10: 229-241.

23. Duhaime AC, Margulies SS, Durham SR, et al. Maturation-dependent response of the piglet brain to scaled cortical impact. *J Neurosurg*. 2000;93:455-462.

24. Haviland J, Russell RI. Outcome after severe non-accidental head injury. *Arch Dis Child*. 1997;77:504-507.

25. Jenny C, Hymel KP, Ritzen A, Reinert SE, Hay TC. Analysis of missed cases of abusive head trauma. *JAMA*. 1999;281:621-626.

26. Ludwig S, Warman M. Shaken baby syndrome: a review of 20 cases. *Ann Emerg Med*. 1984;13:104-107.

27. Johnson DL, Boal D, Baule R. Role of apnea in nonaccidental head injury. *Pediatr Neurosurg*. 1995;23:305-310.

28. Geddes JF, Hackshaw AK, Vowles GH, Nickols CD, Whitwell HL. Neuropathology of inflicted head injury in children. I. Patterns of brain damage. *Brain*. 2001;124(pt 7):1290-1298.

29. Geddes JF, Whitwell HL, Graham DI. Traumatic axonal injury: practical issues for diagnosis in medicolegal cases. *Neuropathol Apply Neurobiol*. 2000;26:105-116.

30. Bonnier C, Nassogne MC, Evrard P. Outcome and prognosis of whiplash shaken infant syndrome; late consequences after a symptom-free interval. *Dev Med Child Neurol*. 1995;37:943-956.

31. Ewing-Cobbs L, Kramer L, Prasad M, et al. Neuroimaging, physical, and developmental findings after inflicted and noninflicted traumatic brain injury in young children. *Pediatrics*. 1998;102: 300-307.

32. Dashti SR, Decker DD, Razzaq A, Cohen AR. Current patterns of inflicted head injury in children. *Pediatr Neurosurg*. 1999;31:302-306.

33. Duhaime AC, Alario AJ, Lewander WJ, et al. Head injury in very young children: mechanisms, injury types, and ophthalmologic

findings in 100 hospitalized patients younger than 2 years of age. *Pediatrics*. 1992;90(pt 1):179-185.

34. Elder JE, Taylor RG, Klug GL. Retinal haemorrhage in accidental head trauma in childhood. *J Paediatr Child Health*. 1991;27:286-289.

35. Johnson DL, Braun D, Friendly D. Accidental head trauma and retinal hemorrhage. *Neurosurgery*. 1993;33:231-235.

36. Christian CW, Taylor AA, Hertle RW, Duhaime AC. Retinal hemorrhages caused by accidental household trauma. *J Pediatr*. 1999;135:125-127.

37. Gleckman AM, Evans RJ, Bell MD, Smith TW. Optic nerve damage in shaken baby syndrome: detection by beta-amyloid precursor protein immunohistochemistry. *Arch Pathol Lab Med*. 2000;124:251-256.

38. Kleinman PK. Radiologic and histopathologic correlates of posterior rib fractures in abused infants: an alternate mechanism of injury. *Pediatr Radiol*. 1987;17:83-91.

39. Kleinman PK, Schlesinger AE. Mechanical factors associated with posterior rib fractures: laboratory and case studies. *Pediatr Radiol*. 1997;27:87-91.

Chapter 3

NEURORADIOLOGY

Marguerite M. Caré, MD

— Manifestations of head injuries in abuse may involve extracranial soft tissues, the cranium, spaces overlying the brain, or the brain itself.

— Often these injuries exhibit patterns suggesting inflicted head trauma.

PARENCHYMAL INJURIES
— Often coexist as devastating injuries in abusive head trauma (AHT).

— More commonly result in death, mental retardation, and permanent neurological impairment.[1-3]

— Can be primary or secondary.

PRIMARY PARENCHYMAL INJURIES
— Include shear-type injuries and parenchymal contusions.

— Are a direct result of traumatic forces inflicted during an abusive event.

— Occur immediately.

— Are less often reversible.

— Are seen infrequently in young patients.

Axonal Injuries
— Diffuse axonal injury is common in patients with severe head trauma,[4] including trauma from high-speed motor vehicle crashes, bicycle accidents, or falls from great heights.

— Widespread traumatic axonal injury is infrequent in AHT except in victims with significant impact injuries.[5-7]

Parenchymal or Cortical Contusions

— May be likened to brain bruises and represent traumatic insults to cortical surfaces and underlying white matter.

— Are common in adults with severe head trauma,[8] less frequent after pediatric head injury,[9,10] and infrequent in child abuse. They are usually seen in slightly older children, not young infants.

— Are clinically less likely than axonal injuries to cause severe neurological outcomes.[4,8]

— Primarily involve superficial gray matter or brain cortex.

— Tend to be multiple and bilateral.

— Are often larger, less defined, and more often hemorrhagic than shear injuries.

— Are usually found in inferior frontal, temporal, and occipital lobes where the brain contacts the irregular floor of the inner table of the skull (**Figure 3-1**).

— Result from localized impacts.

— Are often associated with fractures or scalp hematomas.

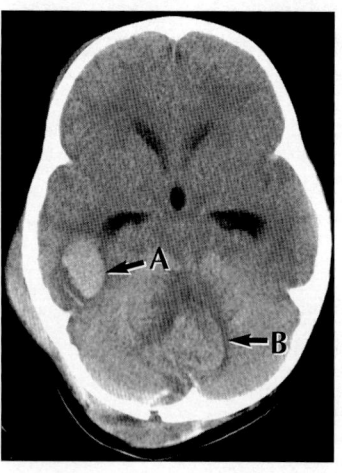

Figure 3-1. *Multifocal cortical contusions in a 3-year-old child with AHT. Axial CT image demonstrates 2 focal areas of acute, cortical contusion. The focal area in the right temporal lobe is well defined, high in attenuation, with some surrounding low attenuation (arrow A). The second focus seen in the superior to mid vermis is slightly more heterogeneous in appearance (arrow B). There is well-defined surrounding edema and complete effacement of the skull base cisterns with evidence of ventricular dilation with enlarged third and temporal horns, as well as some extra-axial acute hemorrhage within the right posterior fossa. A diastatic right occipital bone fracture with extensive overlying swelling is present.*

SECONDARY PARENCHYMAL INJURIES

— Occur in response to primary injuries.[11]

— Include swelling or edema and hypoxia-ischemia.

— Although often seen on initial imaging, secondary injuries can sometimes be reduced by early surgical or medical therapy to decrease overall brain injury.

— In AHT, attempts to treat may be unsuccessful because of delay in seeking care, incomplete and inaccurate histories, or devastating injuries.

— Can lead to severe brain injuries.

Cerebral Edema

— Diffuse brain swelling (edema) after severe head injury is more common in children than adults.[12,13]

— Focal or diffuse swelling may result from, or be associated with, prolonged seizures, direct vascular occlusions, cerebral contusions, diffuse axonal injury, hypoxic-ischemic injuries, and hypoperfusion from shock.[12-14]

— Diffuse cerebral swelling in children (malignant hyperemic cerebral swelling) may result from increased cerebral blood volume and hyperemia.[12]

– Swelling can significantly increase intracranial pressure (ICP) in hours to days, leading to brain herniation or death.[12,13]

— Computed tomography (CT) scans:

1. Show early subtle decreased attenuation within the brain with loss of gray-white matter differentiation.

2. Edema is often diffuse, affecting one or both cerebral hemispheres, but can be focal.

3. There is often progressive effacement of the cortical sulci, ventricles, and basal cisterns that may progress to herniation (**Figure 3-2**).

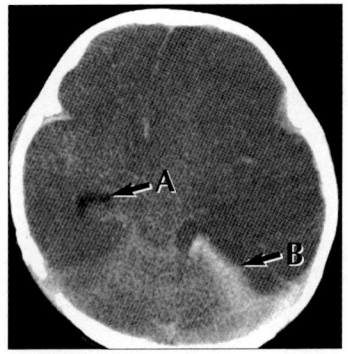

Figure 3-2. Axial CT image of 2½-year-old abused child demonstrates extensive and diffuse cerebral and cerebellar edema with loss of gray-white matter differentiation. There is effacement of the skull base cisterns with early dilation of the right temporal horn (arrow A). There are scattered areas of acute, hyperattenuating intracranial hemorrhage with the largest collection on the left tentorial leaflet (arrow B) and extending along the adjacent left cerebral hemisphere.

4. Ventricles and cisterns may be asymmetrically dilated by herniation and entrapment of cerebrospinal fluid (CSF) spaces.

5. Particular attention should be paid to loss of ambient and quadrigeminal plate cisterns, which are especially sensitive to increased ICP.[15]

6. Progressive edema may cause vascular compression and occlusion with secondary ischemia or infarction.

— Acutely, magnetic resonance imaging (MRI) demonstrates increased signal within affected regions on T2-weighted images.

1. In infants, normal gray-white matter differentiation is easy to visualize on T2-weighted images.

2. With edema, the loss of gray-white matter differentiation on conventional sequences is subtle but often evident.

3. With coexisting ischemia or infarction (cytotoxic edema), edema is readily apparent on diffusion-weighted imaging (DWI).

4. Effacement of the ventricles, cisterns, and cortical sulci will be present.

5. Signs of herniation are well characterized.

HYPOXIC-ISCHEMIC INJURIES
— Often overlap with diffuse cerebral edema processes.

1. The pattern of injury may suggest diffuse hypoperfusion.

2. There is loss of gray-white matter differentiation on imaging but relative preservation of the ventricular sizes and extra-axial spaces (**Figure 3-3**).

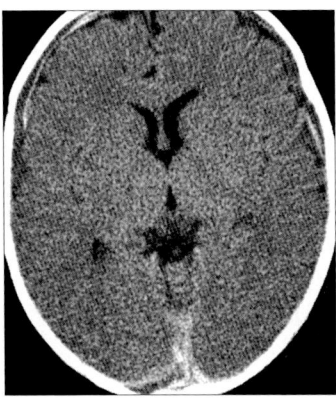

Figure 3-3. *Diffuse hypoxic-ischemic insult or hypoperfusion in a 5-month-old abused infant initially seen with seizure. The axial CT image demonstrates diffuse abnormal low attenuation within the cerebral hemispheres with loss of gray-white matter differentiation. There is some sparing of the left basal ganglia. There is preservation of the subarachnoid and ventricular systems. Scattered areas of subdural hemorrhage are also seen along both cerebral hemispheres. These are mixed in attenuation.*

3. The etiology is unknown, but it is a pattern seen in abuse.

— CT scans:

1. Subtle findings of edema may be seen 2 to 3 hours[11] after initial insult.

2. The initial finding is subtle loss of gray-white matter differentiation in the involved vascular distributions.

3. Extensive injury may involve both cerebral hemispheres.

4. Basal ganglia and cerebellar involvement suggests more prolonged or profound injury.

5. Within several hours, CT scans show better-defined, focal or diffuse low attenuation involving white matter and overlying cortex with further loss of gray-white matter differentiation.

— Injury related to hypoperfusion may not cause effacement of the ventricular system.

1. There is diffuse loss of gray-white matter differentiation as in diffuse edema, but the ventricular size is relatively maintained.

2. Significantly elevated ICP may not develop, so children often are not given steroids.

3. Both diffuse hypoxic-ischemic injury and edema can cause devastating brain injuries (**Figures 3-4-a** and **b**).

— Reversal sign (**Figure 3-5**):

1. Is a distinct radiological finding on CT scan. It is not unique to abuse.[2,16]

2. Is a more profound imaging appearance of diffuse hypoperfusion insult.

3. CT scan shows diffuse, decreased attenuation of cortical gray and white matter with loss of gray-white matter differentiation and relatively increased attenuation in basal ganglia, thalami, brainstem, and cerebellum.

— MRI:

1. Edema is often subtle on conventional magnetic resonance (MR) sequences in young infants because of the normal hyperintense signal of immature, unmyelinated white matter.[14,17]

2. T2-weighted images do not demonstrate well the signal abnormality of the white matter edema but do show loss of gray-white matter differentiation.

3. Advanced imaging sequences, including DWI and MR spectroscopy,[18-21] can readily demonstrate regions of injury and neuronal damage (**Figures 3-6-a, b,** and **c**). These should be included in routine MRI protocol.

— Imaging after acute phase shows profound parenchymal volume loss resulting in devastating neurological outcomes.

EXTRA-AXIAL HEMORRHAGES
Subdural Hematomas
— Are the most commonly described neuroimaging abnormalities in child abuse.

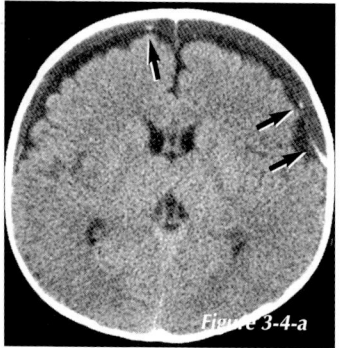 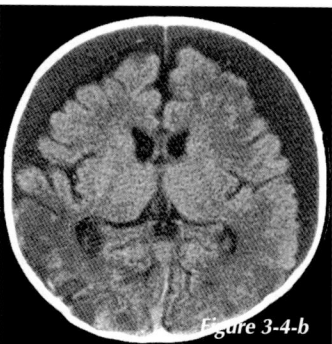

Figure 3-4-a. Diffuse hypoxic-ischemic insult or hypoperfusion in a 4-month-old abused infant. Axial CT image obtained on the date of clinical presentation demonstrates diffuse loss of gray-white matter differentiation with abnormal low attenuation centered in the occipital lobes. There is preservation of the ventricular system and subarachnoid spaces as well as preservation of the basilar and capsular structures. Bilateral, low-attenuation subdural collections with scattered areas of acute hemorrhage (arrows) are also seen within the subdural space.

Figure 3-4-b. Axial CT image obtained 3 weeks following initial presentation demonstrates diffuse and extensive parenchymal volume loss. There has been a significant increase in size in bilateral, low-attenuation subdural collections.

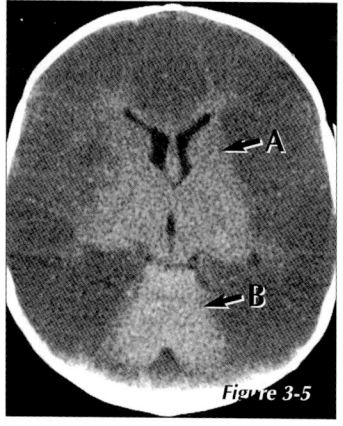

Figure 3-5. Reversal sign in a 2-month-old abused infant. Axial CT image demonstrates diffuse and extensive abnormal attenuation throughout both cerebral hemispheres with loss of gray-white matter differentiation. Although there is loss of differentiation of the basilar and capsular structures, they appear hyperattenuating to the adjacent cerebral hemispheres (arrow A). Also, the cerebellum appears hyperattenuating (arrow B). These findings are the result of a diffuse and extensive hypoxic-ischemic insult.

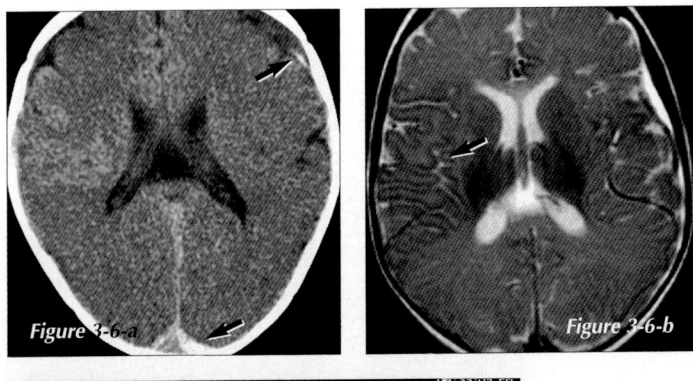

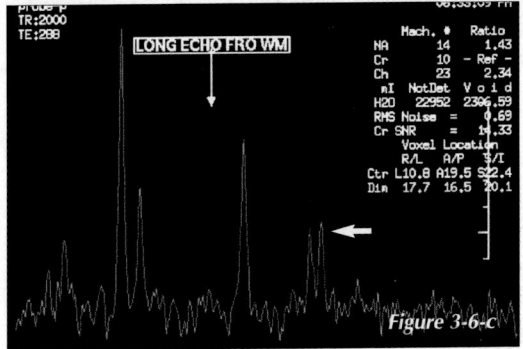

Figures 3-6-a, b, and *c.* Advanced imaging sequences in a 5-month-old abused infant seen with irritability and full anterior fontanel.

Figure 3-6-a. Axial CT image demonstrates a diffuse and extensive hypoxic-ischemic insult with abnormal low attenuation throughout both cerebral hemispheres and loss of gray-white matter differentiation. There is preservation of the subarachnoid space anteriorly with preservation of the lateral ventricles. Scattered areas of acute, hyperattenuating subdural hemorrhage are present (arrows).

Figure 3-6-b. Axial T2-weighted image demonstrates fairly diffuse loss of gray-white matter differentiation with some sparing in the right insular cortex (arrow). The ventricles and subarachnoid spaces are preserved.

Figure 3-6-c. Long echo signal voxel MR spectroscopy from the frontal white matter demonstrates presence of a lactate peak or doublet (arrow). Lactate is present due to the ischemic injury. Ratios and peaks also suggest neuronal loss with cell injury as evidenced by a decrease in N-acetylaspartate, a neuronal marker, and elevation of choline.

— Are often seen with other injury patterns.

— Develop within a potential space between the outer dura mater and the inner pia-arachnoid membrane. This space does not normally contain fluid.

— Rotational and angular forces applied during shaking and shaking with impact cause the brain and cortical vessels to move with respect to the fixed dural sinuses and calvaria, disrupting small cortical arteries or bridging veins and causing bleeding into subdural space.

— Spontaneous subdural hematomas (SDHs) are rarely seen in young infants who are not abused.

1. They may occur following vaginal and cesarean deliveries; in children with coagulation defects or vascular abnormalities; following ventricular shunting; in children with significant parenchymal volume loss or intracranial infections; and in cases of more significant accidental trauma.[9,14,22-24]

2. They are common in AHT.[3,9,10,25]

— Acute SDHs are readily seen on CT scans because of the hyperattenuating appearance of freshly clotted blood (**Figure 3-7**).

1. Large hematomas, hyperacute hemorrhages, and hemorrhages mixed with CSF from dural tears may be more heterogeneous and not show hyperattenuation.

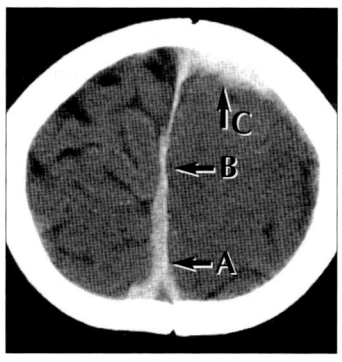

Figure 3-7. Acute subdural hemorrhage on CT scan in a 12-month-old abused infant found unresponsive. Single axial CT image obtained high over the cerebral hemispheres demonstrates acute, high-attenuation interhemispheric subdural hemorrhage (arrows A and B) as well as hemorrhage extending over the high left cerebral convexity (arrow C). There is loss of gray-white matter differentiation in the high cerebral hemispheres with more prominent effacement of the cortical sulci on the left. This is consistent with an extensive, acute brain injury.

2. These collections may appear mixed or even hypoattenuating,[8,11] causing some confusion with cases of rebleeding into chronic subdural collections.

3. The presence of a coexisting acute brain injury or significant mass effect can indicate the age of the injury as these injuries should not be present in cases of simple rebleeding.

— Anatomy:

1. SDHs appear as crescentic collections lying between the skull and brain.

2. The medial margin with the brain is concave.

3. Collections may extend along the entire cerebral convexity and are not confined by the subperiosteal attachment of an adjacent suture.

4. SDHs do not cross the midline because of the falx.

— Small collections:

1. Can be missed on axial CT scan because they may be located over a convexity or near adjacent dense bone.

2. Often exert subtle or no mass effect.

3. May cause minor effacement of adjacent cortical sulci.

— Larger collections:

1. May displace adjacent brain.

2. May cause effacement of ventricles and basal cisterns, midline shift, and other signs of herniation.

— Bilateral and isodense SDHs:

1. May be missed based on symmetry or attenuation, respectively.

2. Viewing CT scan on intermediate windows aids visualization.

3. By postprocessing initial imaging data from routine head CT scan acquired on new multislice CT scanners, image slices as thin as 0.625 mm and multidimensional reconstructed images are available in seconds to minutes and help differentiate subtle abnormalities.

— SDHs adjacent to the posterior interhemispheric fissure:

1. Are characteristic of AHT (**Figure 3-8**).

2. Appear as thickening or increased density of the falx with convex lateral and flattened medial borders.

3. May extend inferiorly to layer on adjacent tentoria[2] or laterally along inner margin of ipsilateral parieto-occipital bone.

— Confusion between dense but normal falx[26] and small SDH is possible.[2]

1. Normal falx:

   A. Can appear asymmetrical or dense, especially in older patients and in young infants and newborns with normally dense dural sinuses.[26]

   B. May appear dense when adjacent brain is abnormally hypo-dense from edema or infarction.[2,27]

2. Acute interhemispheric subarachnoid blood may appear similar,[28] but the blood often extends into the adjacent cortical sulci.

3. MRI is useful when confusion exists because MRI demonstrates signal characteristics of hemorrhage distinct from adjacent dural sinuses or normal but thickened falx.

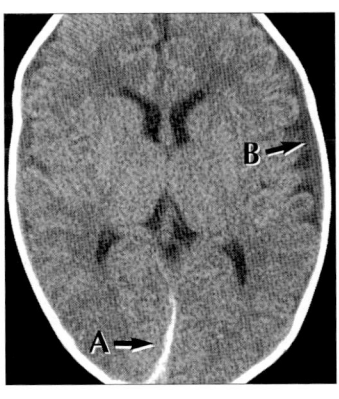

Figure 3-8. *Acute posterior interhemispheric subdural hematoma in a 5-month-old abused infant. Axial CT image demonstrates acute, high-attenuation posterior interhemispheric subdural hemorrhage (arrow A), extending along the right occipital lobe. Although subtle, there is also evidence of a subdural collection with lower attenuation adjacent to the left cerebral hemisphere (arrow B). There is early loss of gray-white matter differentiation in both occipital lobes suggesting acute brain injury.*

A. Acute SDHs are hyperattenuating and gradually (often in the first 2 weeks) become isoattenuating to gray matter, confusing them with the adjacent brain.

1. As they evolve, collections may decrease in size.

2. Collections can also increase in size, especially in patients with devastating brain injuries. As brain volume decreases, the subdural collection increases in size to fill the volume of the calvaria.

3. Hematomas also gradually become more hypoattenuating over a matter of weeks[29] and are often referred to as chronic SDHs.

4. Collections may remain slightly hyperattenuating to CSF.

— CT scan identifies most acute SDHs, but MRI is better to identify subtle collections (**Figures 3-9-a** and **b**).

— The appearance of blood on MRI is complex.

1. Dating hemorrhages on MRI is not reliable.

2. Appearance is influenced by the size of the collection, location, pulse sequence and parameters used, oxidation state of hemoglobin, red blood cell integrity, and field strength of magnet, among other factors.[30-32]

3. MRI is helpful in cases of questionable rebleeds into SDHs.

4. MRI demonstrates the presence of subtle subarachnoid hemorrhages (SAHs) or clots separate from the subdural space and can indicate the presence of significant reinjury.

5. Rebleeding does not cause hemorrhages in the subarachnoid space and should not cause acute brain injuries.

6. Determine the timing of injuries based on MRI studies with caution.[33]

Chronic SDHs

— May be found in infants who have suffered significant previous trauma.

— Are common sequelae in abuse.[34]

— Many children with chronic subdural collections have enlarged or enlarging head circumferences rather than acute injuries.

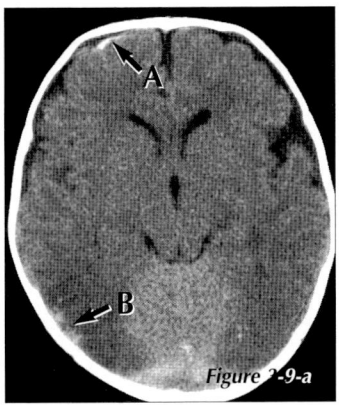 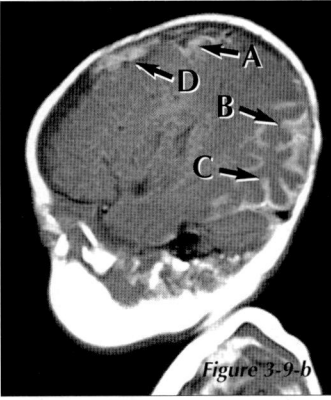

Figures 3-9-a and **b.** *Acute subdural and subarachnoid hemorrhage on CT and MRI scans in a 3-month-old abused infant with seizures. The child sustained a witnessed shaking injury.*

Figure 3-9-a. *Initial axial CT image demonstrates acute high-attenuation extra-axial hemorrhage adjacent to the right frontal lobe (arrow A) with more subtle acute subarachnoid hemorrhage extending into cortical sulci in the region of the right occipital lobe (arrow B). Minimal hemorrhage also is layering on the tentorium. There is acute brain injury with abnormal low attenuation and loss of gray-white matter differentiation predominantly in both posterior temporal and occipital regions.*

Figure 3-9-b. *Sagittal T1-weighted image in the right parasagittal region demonstrates abnormal increased T1 signal layering within the cortical sulci of the right cerebral hemisphere (arrows A, B, and C). Also, there is high-signal subdural hemorrhage high over the right cerebral hemisphere (arrow D).*

— These children may have seizures or signs of developmental delay, lethargy, or failure to thrive.[34]

— The source is often clinically uncertain but presumed traumatic.

— The diagnosis of abuse often relies on finding associated and unexplained skeletal or retinal injuries[35] as well as the history provided.

— Often show varied, complex appearance on imaging (**Figures 3-10-a, b,** and **c**).

1. Septations or membranes may appear to separate the subdural space into multiple compartments. Each compartment may con-

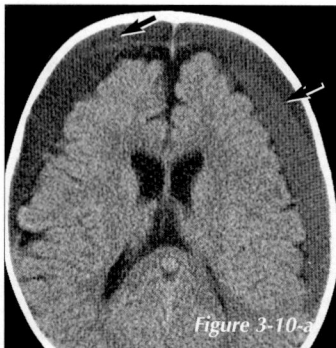

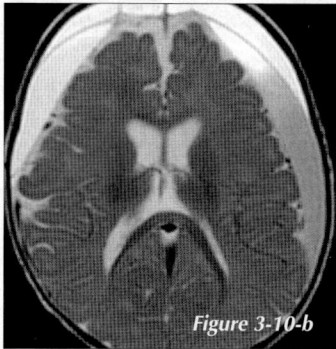

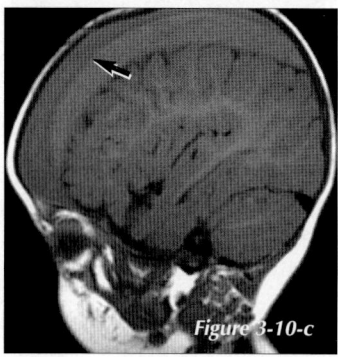

Figures 3-10-a, b, and **c.** Complex, chronic subdural hematomas in a 9-month-old infant suffering from prior abuse.

Figure 3-10-a. Axial CT image demonstrates large, mixed-attenuation subdural collections containing septations (arrows). On the left, the collections demonstrate differing attenuations. All collections remain hyperattenuating to the cerebrospinal fluid in the adjacent subarachnoid space.

Figure 3-10-b. Axial T2-weighted MRI scan demonstrates large bilateral, complicated subdural collections containing septations and different signal intensities. The large collections cause some flattening of the cerebral hemispheres. There is displacement of the cortical veins in the subarachnoid space.

Figure 3-10-c. Sagittal T1-weighted image demonstrates complicated, large subdural collections. The large collection contains a long septation with differing signal intensities on either side (arrow).

tain hemorrhage or fluid of densities or signal characteristics representing different stages of hemorrhage degradation.

2. There may be layering of blood products within the compartments.

3. Rebleeding may occur even with minor or insignificant added trauma.[34,36,37]

— Often cause only localized compression or no mass effect on adjacent brain.

— May be quite large, requiring subdural tapping to reduce size, but should not contribute to acute brain injuries and brain herniation.

— Appearance on CT scan is typically hypoattenuating but can remain slightly hyperattenuating to normal CSF in adjacent subarachnoid spaces and ventricles.

— On MRI, the appearance varies depending on hemorrhagic or protein composition and stage of breakdown of blood products.

— The potential to suggest different ages of hematomas is based on differing signal characteristics or number of bleeding episodes. *CAUTION: Multiple factors affect hemoglobin degradation.*[30-33,38]

— Differentiate chronic SDHs from enlarged subarachnoid spaces in benign macrocrania or the normal large subarachnoid spaces[39,40] by location within the potential subdural space.

1. Fluid is not normal in the subdural space, so collections here are not benign.

2. Not all subdural collections result from abuse.

3. Abnormal fluid collections in the subdural space do not enlarge cortical sulci.

4. Subdural collections displace the cortical veins against the brain surface, whereas vessels will extend through enlarged subarachnoid spaces.[41]

5. Differentiation is more easily made on MRI[42] and ultrasound than CT scan.

6. Chronic sequelae of abuse include chronic SDHs and pathologically enlarged subarachnoid spaces, either from parenchymal volume loss or posttraumatic communicating hydrocephalus. Several findings can coexist.

Benign Macrocrania

— Is also called benign enlargement of subarachnoid spaces,[43] benign subdural collections of infancy,[44,45] benign communicating hydrocephalus,[46] and benign extracerebral fluid collections.[47]

— May cause confusion in abuse.

— Clinically, young infants and children have macrocrania, benign enlargement of subarachnoid spaces, and normal neurological findings.

— Initial imaging findings may be noted around age 3 to 6 months and typically resolve by age 24 to 36 months.

— Parents may report having had larger heads in infancy.

— Enlarged subarachnoid spaces are usually found in a bifrontal location and extend into the anterior interhemispheric fissure.

— They are isoattenuating to CSF within the ventricles, which are usually in the upper normal range or mildly enlarged.

—Enlarged subarachnoid spaces are separated from subdural collections by traversing vessels.

1. In subdural collections, vessels are displaced medially, close to the adjacent brain.

2. This finding is better appreciated on MRI or ultrasound with Doppler sonography through the anterior fontanel (**Figures 3-11 a and b**).[48]

— All young children have larger extra-axial spaces than older children and adults and commonly suffer at least minor household trauma without developing SDHs.

Rebleeding

— Septations or membranes in chronic SDHs may predispose children to repeated bleeding with little or no added trauma.[34,36,37]

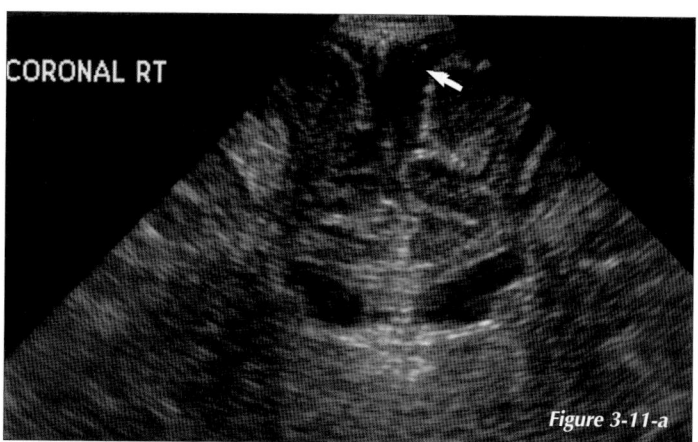

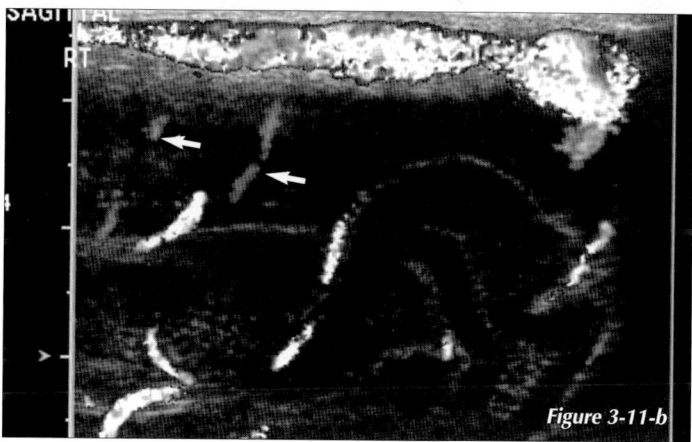

Figures 3-11-a and **b.** Benign macrocrania in a young child with enlarged head circumference.

Figure 3-11-a. Coronal head ultrasound demonstrates mild enlargement of the subarachnoid spaces along the interhemispheric fissure (arrow). There is mild prominence of the lateral ventricles.

Figure 3-11-b. Sagittal ultrasound image demonstrates cortical vessels extending across the enlarged subarachnoid space (arrows).

— Does not occur in remote subdural locations or subarachnoid space.

— With chronic subdural collections, rebleeding may produce mixed-attenuation signal, representing acute hemorrhage superimposed on low-attenuation, chronic SDHs.

— Should not cause acute neurological deterioration.

— Asymptomatic rebleeding is sometimes seen on routine follow-up studies in children with large subdural collections.

— Reinjury is likely in children with chronic SDH who develop new neurological symptoms and evidence of acute hemorrhages and/or parenchymal injuries.

— Confusion may occur in children with hyperacute or actively bleeding mixed-attenuation SDHs.[11,37]

— With fractures, acute mental status change, intracranial mass effect and midline shift, and/or coexistent parenchymal injury, suspect hyperacute bleeding.

— Short-term follow-up images may show hyperacute collections as more homogeneously hyperattenuating and more visible.

Subarachnoid Hemorrhages
— Are a common but often subtle neuroradiological finding in abuse[2,9] (**Figures 3-12-a, b,** and **c**).

— Likely cause is disruption of small cortical vessels after severe acceleration-deceleration forces—similar to the mechanism causing SDHs.

— SAHs and SDHs often coexist in abuse.

— CT scan:

1. Acute SAHs are hyperattenuating or bright compared to the adjacent brain.

2. They are often found high over the cerebral convexities or in the region of the interhemispheric fissure where it conforms to the surface of the brain, extending into the cortical sulci and causing little or no local mass effect.

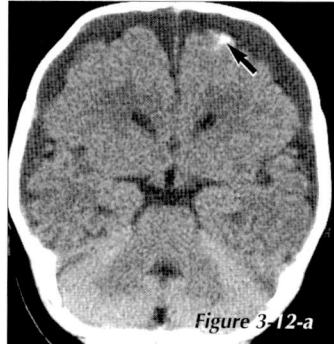

Figure 3-12-a

Figure 3-12-a. *Initial axial CT scan obtained in a child suffering from AHT demonstrates a focal area of high attenuation and acute subarachnoid hemorrhage adjacent to the left frontal lobe (arrow). This hemorrhage extends into the cortical sulci and is separate from low attenuation, but hyperattenuating to cerebrospinal fluid subdural collections extending along both cerebral hemispheres. The presence of acute hemorrhage outside of the subdural space is suggestive of an acute injury and not thought to be from rebleeding into chronic subdural collections.*

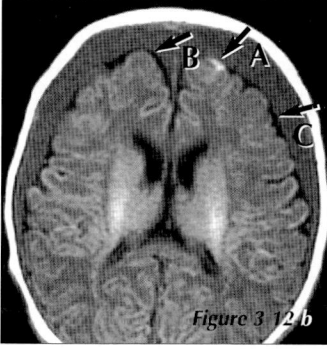

Figure 3-12-b

Figure 3-12-b. *Axial inversion recovery image from a brain MRI scan demonstrates a focal area of increased signal corresponding with the subarachnoid hemorrhage adjacent to the left frontal lobe (arrow A). The MRI scan demonstrates the differentiation between the large subdural collections and the more medial, hypointense subarachnoid space (arrows B and C).*

Figure 3-12-c. *Axial gradient echo image from a brain MRI scan demonstrates a significant "blooming" artifact related to the focal subarachnoid clot in the region of the left frontal lobe (arrow).*

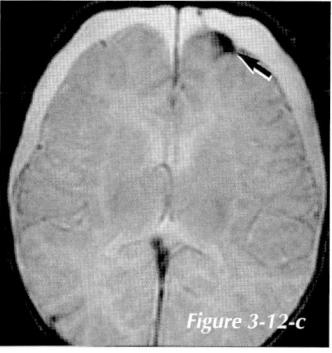

Figure 3-12-c

3. Other common locations are within the basal cisterns and layering along the tentorium.

4. Over days, dense blood becomes less obvious as it degrades and disperses within the subarachnoid space.

5. The subarachnoid space normally contains CSF and is in continuity with the ventricular system, so imaging studies may only demonstrate acute subarachnoid blood for a matter of days because normal CSF is continuously resorbed and produced.

— MRI demonstrates subtle SAHs or clots with the use of gradient echo sequences as well as sagittal and coronal imaging, permitting better visualization of the subarachnoid spaces high over the cerebral convexities.

— Rebleeding into chronic subdural collections does not occur into or cause bleeding in the subarachnoid space.

Epidural Hematomas

— Acute epidural hematomas (EDHs) are uncommon in infants and young children with head injury.[9,10]

— They likely occur from translational or linear forces, such as a direct blow, applied to the calvaria. These forces are similar to those causing fractures or skull deformities.[9,49]

— Most EDHs are associated with fractures.[50]

— May result from arterial or dural venous sinus injuries and may be found within the posterior fossa or supratentorial compartment.[51]

— Delayed or missed diagnosis is associated with high morbidity and mortality.

— May produce a lucid interval lasting more than 24 hours before the child develops deteriorating neurological signs and symptoms[52] as hematoma expansion creates increased mass effect on the adjacent brain.

— Acute EDHs appear as lenticular or biconvex collections adjacent to the inner table of the skull.

— They are typically hyperattenuating on CT scan but may appear heterogeneous if large, actively bleeding, or mixing with CSF from a dural tear (**Figure 3-13**).

— In the posterior fossa, they may appear concave or crescentic.

— They often cause significant mass effect, especially in the infratentorial compartment, where even small collections may significantly compress the brainstem and cause apnea or cardiac demise.

— Smaller EDHs in relatively asymptomatic children are often followed clinically and not evacuated.

1. EDHs age over several days to weeks and become progressively less attenuating.

2. As they mature, the collections often conform to the convexity of the adjacent brain and appear concave.

CRANIAL AND EXTRA-CRANIAL INJURIES

— The presence of bruising, abrasions, scalp hematomas, and edema helps diagnose abuse, but there may be minimal or no external signs of trauma, even with significant intracranial injuries.[27,53]

— Scalp injuries may be evident only at autopsy.[53] Lack of soft tissue swelling does not preclude acute trauma.

— Lack of swelling may result from the child's hemodynamic status or impact against a relatively soft surface.

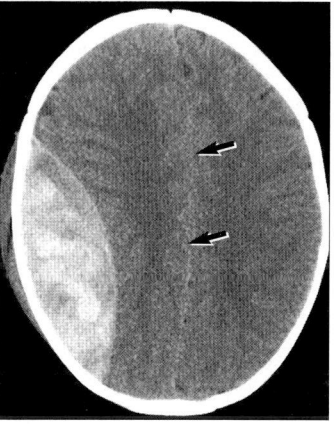

Figure 3-13. *Axial CT image demonstrates a large, biconvex, predominantly high-attenuation hemorrhage in the extra-axial space adjacent to the right cerebral hemisphere. The biconvex appearance is consistent with an epidural hematoma causing significant mass effect on the right cerebral hemisphere with marked right-to-left midline shift of the interhemispheric fissure (arrows).*

— Skull radiographs show soft tissue injuries but are seldom indicated in the evaluation of scalp injuries.

— CT scan:

1. Demonstrates swelling and suspected head injuries.

2. Allows evaluation of the underlying brain.

3. Review of images on intermediate or wide soft tissue window widths allows optimal assessment of extracranial soft tissues.

— Soft tissue swelling:

1. Usually indicates acute events and should prompt a search for underlying fractures or intracranial injuries, especially in young infants.[54]

2. Healing skull fractures do not show radiographic signs of healing (new bone formation and callus), so swelling or lack thereof may help set the age of the fracture.

— Skull fractures caused by abuse are rare; most head injuries are caused by accidents[9,55] (**Figures 3-14-a** and **b**). See Chapter 1, Recognizing Intentional and Unintentional Head Injuries).

— Conventional skull radiographs are best for showing skull fractures.[14]

1. Frontal and lateral skull images are part of a full skeletal series. They are necessary in all young children with suspected abuse.[56]

2. Skull images obtained after CT scans cannot serve as the primary diagnostic imaging step in evaluating suspected head injury.

— Coronal, sagittal, and 3-dimensional (3-D) reformatted images available from initial axial imaging data obtained with routine head CT scan allow better visualization of subtle fractures not always seen on axial view.

— CT imaging is invaluable in assessing depressed or complex skull fractures and identifying acute injuries to the underlying brain.

— Bone scans must be supplemented with conventional skull radiographs.

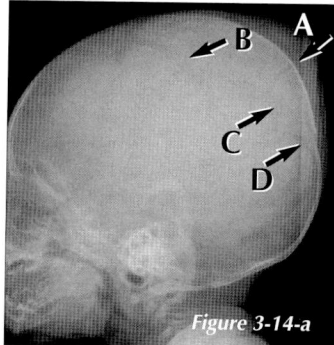

Figure 3-14-a. *Lateral skull radiograph obtained as part of the skeletal survey. The radiograph demonstrates a complex biparietal fracture with a nondisplaced component extending over the convexity (arrow A), and more diastatic component (arrows B, C, and D) extending obliquely through the right parietal bone. The fracture extends into the right coronal and lambdoidal suture.*

Figure 3-14-b. *Single image from the axial CT scan demonstrates acute, extra-axial hemorrhage underlying the complex right parietal bone fracture (arrows A and B) and extending along the posterior interhemispheric fissure (arrows C and D).*

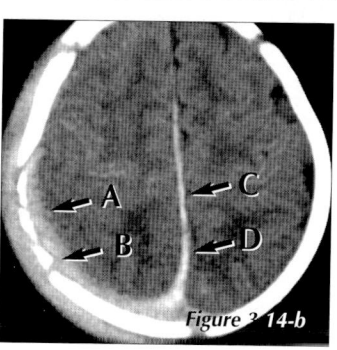

— MRI:

1. Is of limited value in assessing or detecting fractures.

2. Cortical bone lacks signal, so it is easy to miss a fracture causing disruption of the normal signal void.

Advanced MRI

MR Spectroscopy

— Is a noninvasive imaging technique that can be performed with routine MRI.

— Provides an in vivo metabolic profile of an area of the brain.

— Among the primary compounds detected are *N*-acetylaspartate, a neuronal marker; choline, a cell membrane marker; creatine, used as a reference; and lactate, a marker of anaerobic metabolism.

— Is used for acute accidental brain injury[57] and AHT in infants.[58]

— May not alter early hospital course but can suggest prognosis and alter long-term rehabilitative care.

DIFFUSION-WEIGHTED IMAGING

— Is a noninvasive imaging technique that can be performed in conjunction with routine MRI.

— This rapid sequence often requires 60 seconds or less to acquire.

1. Can be used to detect acute focal or global ischemia.

2. Better than conventional MR pulse sequences for early detection of parenchymal ischemia or infarction.[18,19,59]

— Relies on diffusion or motion of water molecules when a magnetic field gradient is applied.

1. Intracellular water accumulates where diffusion is restricted, producing areas of increased signal intensity.[14,59,60]

2. Contribution of the T2 signal in areas of brain injury can "shine through" and complicate interpretation.

3. Apparent diffusion coefficients (ADC), or ADC mapping:

    A. ADC maps are obtained by postprocessing the diffusion data.

    B. They provide a better representation of areas of restricted diffusion or cell injury. These areas will be decreased in signal on the ADC maps.

— Applications:

1. Assess acute ischemia and infarction[61]

2. Demonstrate areas of ischemia within minutes of injury[18,19,62]

3. Differentiate areas of cytotoxic and vasogenic edema[62]

4. Demonstrate ischemic injuries when conventional imaging is difficult to interpret[19,63,64]

TIMING OF INJURIES

— Except in the rare case of expanding EDH with a prolonged lucid interval,[51] abused children or infants sustaining severe parenchymal injuries or fatal head trauma experience an immediate or acute onset of clinical symptoms[1,35,65] that correlates with acute imaging changes.

— Subtle signs of significant brain swelling and infarction from acute injuries can be seen early on CT scans, even within a few hours.[11,65]

— Significant parenchymal abnormalities, including edema and infarction, should not be considered a delayed reaction to a remote traumatic event[65] or caused by simple rebleeding into a chronic SDH.[11]

— Playful, alert infants or young children have not sustained significant, acute injuries that will manifest hours to days later.

— Timing of injuries is best made with a multidisciplinary approach, using a compilation of radiographic studies, physical examination, and historical data.

DIFFERENTIAL DIAGNOSIS

— Before imaging, patients with unsuspected head injury may manifest signs and symptoms that suggest sepsis, infection, seizures, apnea, upper respiratory infections, and failure to thrive.

— A definitive diagnosis of abusive injury is possible[35]:

1.   With characteristic skeletal injuries.

2.   With clearly inflicted soft tissue bruising or burns.

3.   With a combination of acute SDHs, other traumatic brain injuries, and retinal hemorrhages with no reliable clinical history.

— Accidental injury is the most difficult alternative diagnosis to exclude (see Chapter 1, Recognizing Intentional and Unintentional Head Injuries).

— Congenital and acquired coagulopathies in infants and young children may result in intracranial hemorrhage or thrombosis and raise suspicions for abuse.[66,67]

1.   These conditions often involve the brain parenchyma, sometimes in characteristic patterns, and seldom result in large extra-axial hemorrhages.

2.   Acquired coagulopathies may develop after intracranial injury.[24]

3.   Other intracranial disease processes; some metabolic disorders (**Figures 3-15-a** and **b**), specifically glutaricaciduria type I; hemophagocytic lymphohistiocytosis; and perinatal or birth injury rarely may be confused with abuse.

4.   Rarely, osteogenesis imperfecta may manifest as a SDH, though this usually causes confusion with skeletal manifestations of abuse.[68]

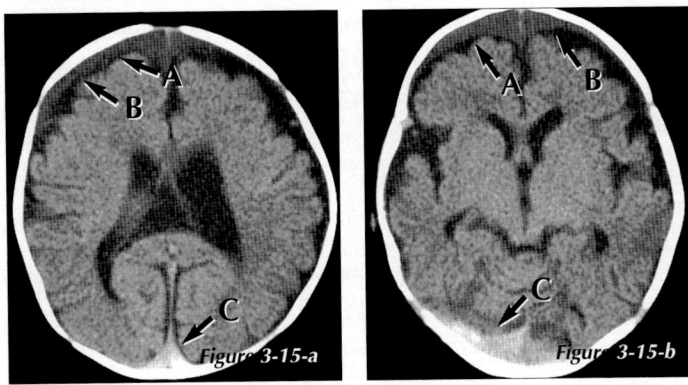

Figure 3-15-a. *A single image from a noncontrast head CT scan demonstrates poor definition of the gray-white matter differentiation and asymmetrical size of the lateral ventricles. The cortical sulci are slightly prominent, as are the subarachnoid spaces. There is a subdural collection (arrows A and B) adjacent to the right frontal lobe and a higher attenuation extra-axial hemorrhage (arrow C) adjacent to the occipital lobes.*

Figure 3-15-b. *An additional image from the same noncontrast CT scan demonstrates prominence of the extra-axial spaces and the cortical sulci involving the cerebrum and the superior cerebellum. In a child with a normal to small head circumference, these findings are suggestive of primary parenchymal volume loss. There are bilateral subdural collections adjacent to the frontal lobes (arrows A and B) that are a higher attenuation than cerebrospinal fluid, as well as more hyperattenuating acute hemorrhage laying on the tentorium (arrow C).*

IMAGING GUIDELINES

— American College of Radiology and other recommendations:

1. Any child aged 5 years or younger with neurological signs and symptoms and a suspicion of abuse should undergo CT evaluation.[69]

2. CT scans are also recommended for children aged 2 years or younger with suspicion of abuse but no focal or neurological findings.[69]

3. Many abused infants are brought for care with supposedly minor or insignificant trauma. AHT should be included in the differential diagnosis of these cases. A lower threshold for obtaining CT scans is needed especially in those younger than 3 months because of the difficulties of making clinical assessments of such young infants.

GUIDELINES FOR CT

—Noncontrast CT is the recommended diagnostic study in the acute setting.[70]

1. CT is readily available, quick, excellent for detecting acute intracranial hemorrhages, and easily performed in acute, traumatic setting.

2. Most modern scanners can obtain a complete set of images in seconds, so the patient's total time in the CT suite is limited to minutes.

3. Acute, life-threatening conditions can be quickly identified.

4. CT scans aid in the limited dating of SDHs.

5. If a hemorrhagic collection is hyperattenuating, bleeding is considered acute.

— CT imaging protocol:

1. Include 5-mm axial images through the entire brain for infants younger than 6 months.

2. Use 5-mm images through the posterior fossa with 10-mm

images through the remaining brain for infants and young children older than 6 months.

3. Thinner imaging through the supratentorial space is often performed.

   A. Thin axial images (3-mm slices) help define questionable extra-axial hemorrhage or parenchymal abnormalities.

   B. On the newer multislice detector CT scanners, even thinner images (0.625 and 1.25 mm) and multiplanar and 3-D images are obtained rapidly by postprocessing the original axial data set.

4. Images should be obtained as conventional axial images because helical acquisitions may cause more artifacts at bony margins or obscure subtle findings.

5. In addition to brain windows, review of images on intermediate windows helps increase conspicuity of acute intracranial hemorrhage.

— Evaluating cranial and extracranial injuries:

1. Review of bone algorithm, scout images, and coronal and sagittal reformatted images when needed, in conjunction with skull radiographs as part of the skeletal survey, aids in evaluating skull fractures and scalp injuries.

2. CT is the modality of choice for imaging acute chest and abdominal injuries that may coexist with skeletal and head injuries.

GUIDELINES FOR MRI
— MRI of the brain is being performed more frequently in suspected abuse.

— Advantages over CT:

1. MRI provides multiplanar imaging, though with CT advances, multiplanar capabilities are less advantageous.

2. MRI provides increased sensitivity for detecting intracranial hemorrhages and parenchymal injuries.[38,71]

3. Detail and visual clarity are increased.[71]

4. MRI readily visualizes small extra-axial hematomas over convexities, in subfrontal and subtemporal locations, and in the posterior fossa.[38]

— Conventional sequences demonstrate subtle SDHs and collections.

— MRI more readily shows some subarachnoid clots that suggest acute insult rather than simple rebleeding into subdural collections.

— Newer techniques increase sensitivity.

— Disadvantages in relation to CT:

1. Less availability, especially in the acute setting

2. Longer imaging times

3. Increased need for sedation

4. Greater difficulty monitoring acutely injured, unstable patients

— MRI should be considered when child abuse is strongly suspected.[72]

— When the CT scan clearly indicates intracranial injury, MRI is not needed, especially acutely.

— With faster MRI and newer technologies, MRI may provide additional information on the extent of parenchymal injuries and the location of extra-axial hemorrhages that may change therapy, prognosis, and rehabilitation.

— When the CT scan is normal or questionably abnormal, MRI may help identify subtle parenchymal injuries or detect subtle SDHs or SAHs.

— Consider MRI for infants and young children in whom there is a high clinical suspicion of abuse or when there are suspicious fractures on the skeletal survey but normal or equivocal findings on the head CT scan.[33,71]

— MRI should be performed when neurological deficits are disproportionate to CT findings.[38]

— MRI through the cervical spine to assess or exclude significant ligamentous injury may be necessary.

— Include T1- and T2-weighted conventional spin echo or fast spin echo images to characterize extra-axial and intraparenchymal hemorrhages and brain injuries.

Spin-Echo Images

Although requiring longer imaging acquisition time, conventional spin echo images are preferred because fast spin echo images are less sensitive in identifying hemorrhages and their breakdown products.

T2-Weighted Images

— In the immature brain, because of high water content, T2-weighted images may not adequately demonstrate some parenchymal injuries.[14,17]

— Bright T2 signal in unmyelinated white matter produces prominent contrast between white matter and the hypointense cortex.

— Established edema is seen as loss of gray-white matter differentiation.

— The first echo often provides enhanced visualization of small extra-axial hemorrhages.

— Like a fluid-attenuated inversion recovery (FLAIR) sequence, this sequence somewhat "suppresses" the bright signal of CSF, allowing visualization of small collections.

T1-Weighted Images

— Obtain T1-weighted images, and especially heavily T1-weighted images using inversion recovery techniques, in all children younger than 1 year.

— This sequence allows better evaluation of the normal myelination pattern.

— Gradient echo sequences should be part of the routine trauma imaging protocol and are particularly useful in abuse cases because of the enhanced sensitivity to demonstrating susceptibility artifact from blood products.[11]

— Areas of remote parenchymal hemorrhage or extra-axial clot demonstrate "blooming artifact" with larger areas of extreme hypointensity.

— Larger, more chronic hematomas are not often uniformly markedly hypointense, but they may contain small areas of clot suggesting prior hemorrhage.

FLAIR Imaging

— Attenuates CSF signal.

— Often provides increased conspicuity of extra-axial collections and some parenchymal injuries.

— In young infants, FLAIR imaging may not detect some nonhemorrhagic parenchymal injuries because of high water content in the immature, unmyelinated brain.

— It is invaluable in children older than 1 year to define parenchymal injuries and extra-axial collections.

MR Spectroscopy and DWI

— Better define parenchymal injuries, even when conventional MRI appears normal.

— Should be used routinely in cases of suspected AHT.

OTHER IMAGING MODALITIES

Ultrasound

— The ability to see posterior fossa structures, the peripheral cortex, and small extracerebral collections and spaces is limited.

— Provides no benefit in evaluating acute intracranial injuries in abuse.[33]

— Can be used in nonacute settings in young infants to evaluate the brain and distinguish prominent subarachnoid spaces from subdural collections in macrocephaly.[48]

Skeletal Survey

— Is indicated in suspected abuse to detect clinically occult skeletal fractures.[69]

— Occult fractures are less common in children aged 2 to 3 years or older, so skeletal surveys may not be needed.

— Suspicious extracranial skeletal injuries include rib fractures, classic metaphyseal lesions (corner or bucket-handle fractures), scapular fractures, multiple fractures, and fractures of various ages.[73]

— Skeletal survey guidelines suggested by the American College of Radiology for children with suspected physical abuse:

1. Obtain a separate radiographic exposure of each anatomical region from the anteroposterior and/or posteroanterior views[56] (**Table 3-1**).

2. The axial skeleton should be imaged in 2 projections, and at least frontal views of all extremities should be obtained. An emerging trend in current practice is to include 2 oblique views of the chest as well as to assess for posterior rib fractures.

3. Use more views as needed to document or confirm suspicious sites of injury.[56]

4. Do follow-up surveys 2 weeks after the initial examination to help define fractures and demonstrate healing fractures.[74]

Table 3-1. Complete Skeletal Survey

Appendicular Skeleton	Axial Skeleton
— Arms (AP)	— Thorax (AP and lateral), to include thoracic spine and ribs
— Forearms (AP)	
— Hands (PA)	— AP abdomen, lumbosacral spine, and bony pelvis
— Thighs (AP)	
— Legs (AP)	— Lumbar spine (lateral)
— Feet (PA) or (AP)	— Cervical spine (AP and lateral)
	— Skull (frontal and lateral)

Reprinted with permission of the Amercian College of Radiology,[56] Reston, Virginia. No other representation of this material is authorized without express, written permission from the American College of Radiology.

Bone Scans
— May be performed if urgent evaluation for occult injuries is needed (eg, in cases in which child placement is an issue).

— Follow-up skeletal surveys are used more often so bone scans are not frequently performed.

DOCUMENTATION
— Be aware of all historical and clinical data.

— Communicate directly with the referring physician.

— Provide clear, comprehensive documentation.

1. The radiology report is part of a patient's medical record, which is a legal document.

2. The medical record is a source of information to health care professionals and public agencies and may be subpoenaed.

3. The medical record can be reviewed before a physician testifies in court, which may not occur for months or years after the incident.

4. Adequate documentation may eliminate the need for physician testimony.

5. Data introduced in court that is not found in the initial medical report may be judged inadmissible.

— Clearly write or type all medical records and radiology reports.

— The reporting physician's signature; the child's name and another means of identifying the child (medical record number); type of examination; date of examination[75]; and a concise, detailed report of all definite and suspected sites of injuries should be included.[56]

— Convey a subjective but professional opinion of suspected child abuse to referring physicians and in the written radiology report.[56]

— The radiology report guides primary physicians in choosing additional imaging to further define abnormalities or look for unsuspected injuries.[75] These may include initial and repeated skeletal surveys, CT or MRI, or bone scans.

— Ensure positive radiographs or imaging studies are properly sequestered in the department so they can be accessed as needed.

— Digital imaging:

1. Images can be brought to the courtroom setting on laptop computers or transported on discs.

2. They are often easier to display and easier for the judge and jury to visualize, permitting enlargement, labeling, and displays for comparison with normal imaging.

REFERENCES

1. Gillis EE, Nelson MD Jr. Cerebral complications of nonaccidental head injury in childhood. *Pediatr Neurol.* 1998;19:119-128.

2. Cohen RA, Kaufman RA, Myers PA, Towbin RB. Cranial computed tomography in the abused child with head injury. *AJR Am J Roentgenol.* 1986;146:97-102.

3. Zimmerman RA, Bilaniuk LT, Bruce D, Schut L, Uzzell B, Goldberg HI. Computed tomography of craniocerebral injury in the abuse child. *Radiology.* 1979;130:687-690.

4. Gentry LR, Godersky JC, Thompson B. MR imaging of head trauma: review of the distribution and radiopathologic features of traumatic lesions. *AJR Am J Roentgenol.* 1988;150:663-672.

5. Geddes JF, Hackshaw AK, Vowles GH, Nickols CD, Whitwell HL. Neuropathology of inflicted head injury in children. I. Patterns of brain injury. *Brain.* 2001;124(pt 7):1290-1298.

6. Geddes JF, Vowles GH, Hackshaw AK, Nickols CD, Scott IS, Whitwell HL. Neuropathology of inflicted head injury in children. II. Microscopic brain injury in infants. *Brain.* 2001; 124(pt 7):1299-1306.

7. Shannon P, Smith CR, Deck J, Ang LC, Ho M, Becker L. Axonal injury and the neuropathology of shaken baby syndrome. *Acta Neuropathol (Berl).* 1998;95:625-631.

8. Gentry LR. Imaging of closed head injury. *Radiology.* 1994;191:1-17.

9. Duhaime AC, Alario AJ, Lewander WJ, et al. Head injury in very young children: mechanisms, injury types, and ophthalmologic findings in 100 hospitalized patients younger than 2 years of age. *Pediatrics.* 1992;90(pt 1):179-185.

10. Merten DF, Osborne DR, Radkowski MA, Leonidas JC. Craniocerebral trauma in the child abuse syndrome: radiological observations. *Pediatr Radiol.* 1984;12:272-277.

11. Barnes PD, Robson CD. CT findings in hyperacute nonaccidental brain injury. *Pediatr Radiol.* 2000;30:74-81.

12. Zimmerman RA, Bilaniuk LT, Bruce D, Dolinskas C, Obrist W, Kuhl D. Computed tomography of pediatric head trauma: acute general cerebral swelling. *Radiology.* 1978;126:403-408.

13. Bruce DA, Alavi A, Bilaniuk L, Dolinskas C, Obrist W, Uzzell B. Diffuse cerebral swelling following head injuries in children: the syndrome of "malignant brain edema." *J Neurosurg.* 1981;54:170-178.

14. Chen CY, Zimmerman RA, Rorke LB. Neuroimaging in child abuse: a mechanism-based approach. *Neuroradiology.* 1999;41:711-722.

15. Ball WS, ed. *Pediatric Neuroradiology.* New York, NY: Lippincott-Raven; 1997.

16. Han BK, Towbin RB, De Courten-Myers G, McLaurin RL, Ball WS Jr. Reversal sign on CT: effect of anoxic/ischemic cerebral injury in children. *AJR Am J Roentgenol.* 1990;154:361-368.

17. Zimmerman RA, Bilaniuk LT. Pediatric head trauma. *Neuroimaging Clin N Am.* 1994;4:349-366.

18. Suh DY, Davis PC, Hopkins KL, Fajman NN, Mapstone TB. Nonaccidental pediatric head injury: diffusion-weighted imaging findings. *Neurosurgery.* 2001;49:309-318, 318-320 [discussion].

19. Biousse V, Suh DY, Newman NJ, Davis PC, Mapstone T, Lambert SR. Diffusion-weighted magnetic resonance imaging in Shaken Baby Syndrome. *Am J Ophthalmol.* 2002;133:249-255.

20. Garnett MR, Blamire AM, Rajagopalan B, Styles P, Cadoux-Hudson TA. Evidence for cellular damage in normal-appearing white matter correlates with injury severity in patients following traumatic brain injury: a magnetic resonance spectroscopy study. *Brain.* 2000;123(pt 7):1403-1409.

21. Sinson G, Bagley LJ, Cecil KM, et al. Magnetization transfer imaging and proton MR spectroscopy in the evaluation of axonal injury: correlation with clinical outcome after traumatic brain injury. *AJNR Am J Neuroradiol.* 2001;22:143-151.

22. Aoki N. Chronic subdural hematoma in infancy. Clinical analysis of 30 cases in the CT era. *J Neurosurg.* 1990;73:201-205.

23. Aoki N, Masuzawa H. Infantile acute subdural hematoma. Clinical analysis of 26 cases. *J Neurosurg.* 1984;61:273-280.

24. Hymel KP, Abshire TC, Luckey DW, Jenny C. Coagulopathy in pediatric abusive head trauma. *Pediatrics.* 1997;99:371-375.

25. Hymel KP, Rumack CM, Hay TC, Strain JD, Jenny C. Comparison of intracranial computed tomographic (CT) findings in pediatric abusive and accidental head trauma. *Pediatr Radiol.* 1997;27:743-747.

26. Osborn AG, Anderson RE, Wing SD. The false falx sign. *Radiology.* 1980;134:421-425.

27. Feldman KW, Brewer DK, Shaw DW. Evolution of the cranial computed tomography scan in child abuse. *Child Abuse Negl.* 1995;18:307-314.

28. Dolinskas CA, Zimmerman RA, Bilaniuk LT. A sign of subarachnoid bleeding on cranial computed tomograms of pediatric head trauma patients. *Radiology.* 1978;126:409-411.

29. Bergstrom M, Ericson K, Levander B, Svendsen P, Larsson S. Variation with time of the attenuation values of intracranial hematomas. *J Comput Assist Tomogr.* 1977;1:57-63.

30. Gomori JM, Grossman RI, Yu-Ip C, Asakura T. NMR relaxation times of blood: dependence on field strength, oxidation state, and

cell integrity. *J Comput Assist Tomogr.* 1987;11:684-690.

31. Zyed A, Hayman LA, Bryan RN. MR imaging of intracerebral blood: diversity in the temporal pattern at 0.5 and 1.0 T. *AJNR Am J Neuroradiol.* 1991;12:469-474.

32. Bradley WG Jr. MR appearance of hemorrhage in the brain. *Radiology.* 1993;189:15-26.

33. Ball WS Jr. Nonaccidental craniocerebral trauma (child abuse): MR imaging. *Radiology.* 1989;173:609-610.

34. Parent AD. Pediatric chronic subdural hematoma: a retrospective comparative analysis. *Pediatr Neurosurg.* 1992;18:266-271.

35. Duhaime AC, Christian CW, Rorke LB, Zimmerman RA. Nonaccidental head injury in infants—the "shaken baby syndrome." *N Engl J Med.* 1998;338:1822-1829.

36. McLone D. Ultrastructure of subdural membranes in children. In: *Concepts in Pediatric Neurosurgery.* Vol 1. New York, NY: Karger; 1981:174-187.

37. Sargent S, Kennedy JG, Kaplan JA. "Hyperacute" subdural hematoma: CT mimic of recurrent episodes of bleeding in the setting of child abuse. *J Forensic Sci.* 1996;41:314-316.

38. Sato Y, Yuh WT, Smith WL, Alexander RC, Kao SC, Ellerbroek CJ. Head injury in child abuse: evaluation with MR imaging. *Radiology.* 1989;173:653-657.

39. Kleinman PK, Zito JL, Davidson RI, Raptopoulos V. The subarachnoid spaces in children: normal variations in size. *Radiology.* 1983;147:455-457.

40. Prassopoulos P, Cavouras D. CT evaluation of normal CSF spaces in children: relationship to age, gender and cranial size. *Eur J Radiol.* 1994;18:22-25.

41. McCluney KW, Yeakley JW, Fenstermacher MJ, Baird SH, Bonmati CM. Subdural hygroma versus atrophy on MR brain scans: "the cortical vein sign." *AJNR Am J Neuroradiol.* 1992;13:1335-1339.

42. Wilms G, Vanderschueren G, Demaerel PH, et al. CT and MR in infants with pericerebral collections and macrocephaly: benign enlargement of the subarachnoid spaces versus subdural collections. *AJNR Am J Neuroradiol.* 1993;14:855-860.

43. Ment LR, Duncan CC, Geehr R. Benign enlargement of the subarachnoid spaces in the infant. *J Neurosurg.* 1981;54:504-508.

44. Robertson WC Jr, Chun RW, Orrison WW, Sackett JF. Benign subdural collections of infancy. *J Pediatr.* 1979;94:382-386.

45. Briner S, Bodensteiner J. Benign subdural collections of infancy. *Pediatrics.* 1981;67:802-804.

46. Kendall B, Holland I. Benign communicating hydrocephalus in children. *Neuroradiology.* 1981;21:93-96.

47. Hamza M, Bodensteiner JB, Noorani PA, Barnes PD. Benign extracerebral fluid collections: a cause of macrocrania in infancy. *Pediatr Neurol.* 1987;3:218-221.

48. Chen CY, Chou TY, Zimmerman RA, Lee CC, Chen FH, Faro SH. Pericerebral fluid collection: differentiation of enlarged subarachnoid spaces from subdural collections with color Doppler US. *Radiology.* 1996;201:389-392.

49. Ommaya AK, Gennarelli TA. Cerebral concussion and traumatic unconsciousness. Correlation of experimental and clinical observations of blunt head injuries. *Brain.* 1974;97:633-654.

50. Shugerman RP, Paez A, Grossman DC, Feldman KW, Grady MS. Epidural hemorrhage: is it abuse? *Pediatrics.* 1996;97:664-668.

51. Schutzman SA, Barnes PD, Mantello M, Scott RM. Epidural hematomas in children. *Ann Emerg Med.* 1993;22:535-541.

52. Choux M, Grisoli F, Peragut JC. Extradural hematomas in children. 104 cases. *Childs Brain.* 1975;1:337-347.

53. Duhaime AC, Gennarelli TA, Thibault LE, Bruce DA, Margulies SS, Wiser R. The shaken baby syndrome. A clinical, pathological, and biomechanical study. *J Neurosurg.* 1987;66:409-415.

54. Schutzman SA, Barnes P, Duhaime AC, et al. Evaluation and management of children younger than two years old with apparently minor head trauma: proposed guidelines. *Pediatrics*. 2001;107: 983-993.

55. Leventhal JM, Thomas SA, Rosenfield NS, Markowitz RI. Fractures in young children. Distinguishing child abuse from unintentional injuries. *Am J Dis Child*. 1993;147:87-92.

56. American College of Radiology. Skeletal surveys in children. *ACR Practice Guidelines* [serial online]. January 1, 2002; Res 31:107-111. Available at: http://www.acr.org. Accessed August 3, 2005.

57. Holshouser BA, Ashwal S, Luh GY, et al. Proton MR spectroscopy after acute central nervous system injury: outcome prediction in neonates, infants, and children. *Radiology*. 1997;202:487-496.

58. Haseler LJ, Arcinue E, Danielsen ER, Bluml S, Ross BD. Evidence from proton magnetic resonance spectroscopy for a metabolic cascade of neuronal damage in shaken baby syndrome. *Pediatrics*. 1997;99:4-14.

59. Warach S, Dashe JF, Edelman RR. Clinical outcome in ischemic stroke predicted by early diffusion-weighted and perfusion magnetic resonance imaging: a preliminary analysis. *J Cereb Blood Flow Metab*. 1996;16:53-59.

60. Chien D, Kwong KK, Gress DR, Buonanno FS, Buxton RB, Rosen BR. MR diffusion imaging of cerebral infarction in humans. *AJNR Am J Neuroradiol*. 1992;13:1097-1102, 1103-1105.

61. Ito J, Marmarou A, Barzo P, Fatouros P, Corwin F. Characterization of edema by diffusion-weighted imaging in experimental traumatic brain injury. *J Neurosurg*. 1996;84:97-103.

62. Hanstock CC, Faden AI, Bendall MR, Vink R. Diffusion-weighted imaging differentiates ischemic tissue from traumatized tissue. *Stroke*. 1994;25:843-848.

63. Cowan FM, Pennock JM, Hanrahan JD, Manji KP, Edwards AD. Early detection of cerebral infarction and hypoxic ischemic en-

cephalopathy in neonates using diffusion-weighted magnetic resonance imaging. *Neuropediatrics*. 1994;25:172-175.

64. Beaulieu C, D'Arceuil H, Hedehus M, de Crespigny A, Kastrup A, Moseley ME. Diffusion-weighted magnetic resonance imaging: theory and potential applications to child neurology. *Semin Pediatr Neurol*. 1999;6:87-100.

65. Willman KY, Bank DE, Senac M, Chadwick DL. Restricting the time of injury in fatal inflicted head injuries. *Child Abuse Negl*. 1997;21:929-940.

66. Yoffe G, Buchanan GR. Intracranial hemorrhage in newborn and young infants with hemophilia. *J Pediatr*. 1988;113:333-336.

67. Dietrich AM, James CD, King DR, Ginn-Pease ME, Cecalupo AJ. Head trauma in children with congenital coagulation disorders. *J Pediatr Surg*. 1994;29:28-32.

68. Tokora K, Nakajima F, Yamataki A. Infantile chronic subdural hematoma with local protrusion of the skull in a case of osteogenesis imperfecta. *Neurosurgery*. 1988;22:595-598.

69. American College of Radiology. ACR appropriateness criteria. *Radiology*. 2000;215(suppl):805-809.

70. Marray JG, Gean AD, Evans SJ. Imaging of acute head injury. *Semin Ultrasound CT MR*. 1996;17:185-205.

71. Alexander RC, Schor DP, Smith WL Jr. Magnetic resonance imaging of intracranial injuries from child abuse. *J Pediatr*. 1986; 109:975-979.

72. Nimkin K, Kleinman PK. Imaging of child abuse. *Pediatr Clin N Am*. 1997;44:615-635.

73. Kleinman PK. *Diagnostic Imaging of Child Abuse*. 2nd ed. St. Louis, Mo: Mosby; 1998.

74. Kleinman PK, Nimkin K, Spevak MR, et al. Follow-up skeletal surveys in suspected child abuse. *AJR Am J Roentgenol*. 1996;167: 893-896.

75. American College of Radiology. Communication: diagnostic radiology. *ACR Practice Guidelines* [serial online]. January 1, 2002; Res 50:5-7. Available at: http://www.acr.org. Accessed August 3, 2005.

NEUROSURGERY

Gary L. Hedlund, DO

Peter Kan, MD

Michael D. Partington, MD, FACS, FAAP

Marion L. Walker, MD

SCALP TRAUMA

SCALP LACERATION

— The simplest form of head injury potentially requiring neurosurgical intervention is the scalp laceration.

— Most are repaired in the emergency department by physicians or general or pediatric surgeons.

— More extensive injuries are managed operatively by neurosurgeons and/or plastic surgeons, especially when large areas of the scalp, degloving injuries, facial trauma, and burns are involved.

CEPHALOHEMATOMA

— Can occur after normal birth or later trauma.

— Located subperiosteally, it is usually confined to a single skull bone and does not cross sutures.

— May accompany skull fracture, but can also be generated by skull deformation, which strips the periosteum off the bone.

— Direct intervention is seldom required because the periosteum tamponades hemorrhage.

— Infection elsewhere in the body can seed the hematoma. Aspiration may be required for diagnosis, culture, and treatment.

— Calcification is a rare late complication, which occurs because the periosteum is the primary generator of bone and can form a calcified rim if it does not resorb.

1. This is largely a cosmetic concern.

2. Treatment, if needed, consists of drilling the abnormal calcified rim down to the level of the normal outer table.

SUBGALEAL HEMATOMA

— Occurs under superficial layers of the scalp.

— Generally signifies injury to an underlying venous sinus.

— Most are related to birth trauma, particularly vacuum extraction.

— The bleeding is not contained by the periosteum. The blood accumulates in a potential space that encompasses the entire scalp and is contiguous with subcutaneous tissues of the chest and abdomen. The large extent of this space, in addition to the fact that the sagittal sinus conveys nearly all of the brain's blood return toward the heart, creates circumstances that can be catastrophic.

— Is often associated with fractures, usually crossing a sinus transversely.

— Management:

1. Hinges on the early recognition of ongoing exsanguination, institution of aggressive volume resuscitation, and correction of coagulopathy.

2. Surgical repair or tamponade of the sinus injury is possible, but only if prompt neurosurgical consultation is available and resuscitation is successful.

SKULL FRACTURE

Fractures are classified according to the portion of the skull involved (basal vs vault), integrity of the overlying skin (open vs closed), and degree of displacement (linear vs depressed)

BASILAR SKULL FRACTURES (FRACTURES OF THE SKULL BASE)

— Are less common in infants than in older children.

— Are often caused by static load mechanism.

— Many are asymptomatic but are diagnosed because of imaging studies or ecchymosis around orbits or ears.

— If symptomatic, a cerebrospinal fluid (CSF) leak, cranial nerve deficit, or both are usually found.

— Most CSF leaks resolve spontaneously after bed rest.

— Persistent leaks require lumbar drain or open surgery.

— Surgical decompression of injured cranial nerves has not been conclusively shown to aid recovery.[1]

FRACTURES OF THE SKULL VAULT
— Usually involve the parietal bone because of the relatively large surface area of the bone itself and maximal transverse width of the vault (at parietal eminences), making this the largest target for potential impact injury.

— A simple nondisplaced linear fracture does not require added treatment.

— If there is an overlying laceration, this is considered an open linear fracture. Typically, only repair of the laceration is required.

— Gross contamination may require cleansing in the operating room, depending on the age and cooperation of the child.

GROWING SKULL FRACTURE (LEPTOMENINGEAL CYST)
— Is defined as a linear fracture that enlarges over time (**Figures 4-1-a** and **b**).

— It is caused by the combination of a rapidly growing brain with a skull fracture and an underlying dural tear.

— Most occur in first 2 years of life.

— It is more common in abusive than accidental head trauma because abusive skull fractures are often larger and more complex.

— It is not unique to or diagnostic of inflicted trauma.

— Management is surgical; there is no evidence of natural reversal.

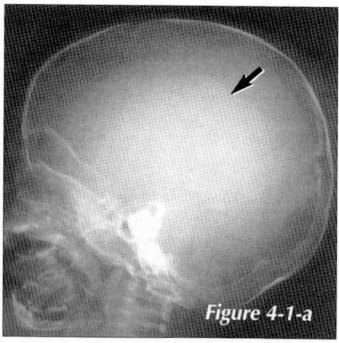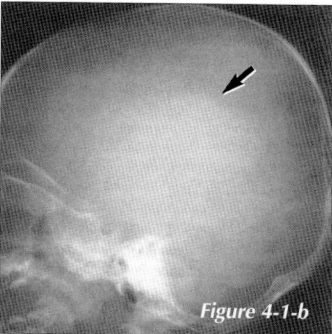

Figure 4-1-a. *Lateral radiograph of the skull of a 6-month-old infant who was accidentally dropped from an adult's arms to a hard-surface floor shows a large parietal fracture (arrow).*

Figure 4-1-b. *Obtained 6 weeks later; not only has the fracture not healed (arrow), but it is considerably wider at its midpoint.*

— Surgery:

1.   Consists of a craniotomy that encompasses bone defect and dural defect, which is usually larger because the dura mater tends to retract beyond the fracture's edge.

2.   The dura mater is patched and the bone replaced, taking care to reshape the bone so the existing defect is over intact native dura mater, which then permits healing.

DEPRESSED FRACTURES

— Are managed according to fracture location, associated injuries, cosmetic significance, and integrity of overlying tissues (**Figures 4-2-a and b**).

— Historically, fractures depressed by full skull thickness or greater have been elevated to reduce the risk of posttraumatic epilepsy, but this approach is not supported by recent evidence.

— If the fracture overlies an associated injury that requires surgery, incorporate fracture repair in craniotomy.

1.   Remove the area of depression as part of opening.

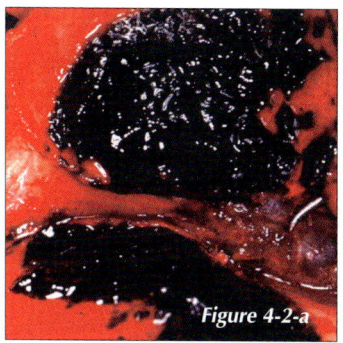 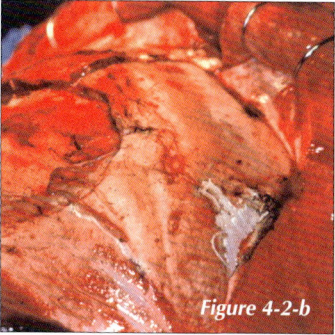

Figure 4-2-a. *A significant amount of epidural blood overlying the dura mater and underneath the bone flap.*

Figure 4-2-b. *Large depressed skull fracture overlying the epidural hematoma.*

2. Realign and replace bone fragments.

    A. Secure bone fragments with suture, wire, metal plates and screws, or absorbable plating systems.

    B. Permanent, rigid fixation systems are not needed. Bones of the cranial vault only need to be held in place while healing.

    C. Wire and metal plate systems can migrate in the growing brain and skull, so absorbable systems are preferred in infants.[2]

— If surgery for an associated injury is not indicated, the choice is based on the visibility of the fractures.

1. A large visible depression on the forehead merits surgical repair.

2. A smaller, partial-thickness depression under hair-bearing scalp may be permitted to remodel over time.

3. If the scalp is open, repair both in the operating room, especially if the integrity of the dura mater is questionable.[3]

PING-PONG FRACTURES
— Are a type of depressed fracture seen exclusively in infants.

— The appearance is similar to indentations caused by pressure applied to a table tennis ball.

— They result from a focal impactor being applied to the head.

— The fracture may "pop out" because of normal underlying bone pressure.

— Conservative management may be appropriate.[4]

— Surgical management involves elevating the fracture fragments.

EPIDURAL HEMATOMA

— An epidural hematoma (EDH) results from bleeding between the dura mater and the skull.

— It is a common intracranial injury of childhood, but it is seen more with accidental head injury (**Figure 4-3**).

— Skull fracture often accompanies an EDH, so management options may need to be based on concern for both injuries.

— The management is specific to the source of bleeding found after computed tomography (CT) imaging.

SMALL EDH

— Generally does not produce midline shift.

— Is usually related to an overlying skull fracture.

— When identified in a conscious, neurologically intact patient, observe in the hospital.

1. Admit the child to the intensive care unit (ICU) or similar setting for close observation.

2. Repeat CT scan in 6 to 12 hours and possibly the next day.

— If the hematoma increases, especially with increased intracra-

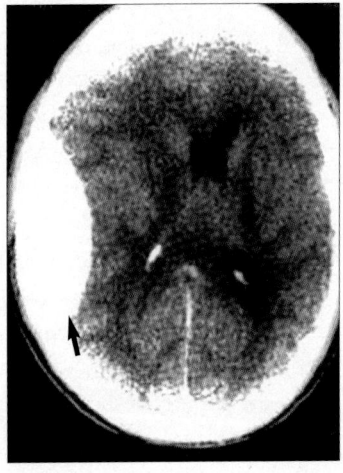

Figure 4-3. *Acute right-sided epidural hematoma (arrow) on CT scan of 3-year-old girl reported to have fallen from the couch.*

nial pressure (ICP) or new neurological deficits, remove the hematoma surgically.

EDH ASSOCIATED WITH DURAL SINUS INJURY

— Is potentially difficult to manage surgically.

— Lesions are identified on CT scan by their proximity to a sinus. The lesions can be large.

— Lesions are often tamponaded by the brain and dura mater.

— If the child is not clinically harmed by its presence, follow the lesion with serial imaging.

— Neurosurgeons need to recognize the likelihood of sinus injury and the high risk of massive blood loss when the clot is removed.

— In infants, bleeding from a dural sinus may cause exsanguination if blood is not immediately available and the surgeon is not prepared to control the bleeding.

EDH CAUSED BY ARTERIAL BLEEDING

— Is more likely to require surgery.

— Is classically associated with a "lucid interval" but can cause immediate coma or no loss of consciousness.

— Infants:

1. Initial signs or symptoms are related to shock from large hematoma volume.

2. Arterial injury is usually to the middle meningeal artery or its branches.

3. The posterior branch can be injured in the parietal region with or without fracture.

— In older children, the injury often relates to a middle fossa fracture.

— Surgery:

1. Is undertaken in patients with a decreased level of consciousness, focal deficits referable to the clot, evidence of herniation, or imaging evidence of clot expansion.

2. The craniotomy is centered over the clot and presumed source of bleeding; the hematoma is evacuated, and the source of bleeding is controlled.

3. Children with EDH usually do well if surgery is timely.[5]

SUBDURAL HEMATOMA

— A subdural hematoma (SDH) in infants is most often associated with shaken baby syndrome.

— In accidental injuries, it usually represents an impact injury.

— Surgery is based on principles similar to those for EDH.

— The features of SDH after intentional injury differ significantly from those of accidental injuries.

SDH IN ABUSIVE HEAD INJURY

— SDH is typically part of global injury in which potentially severe brain injury accompanies hematoma and becomes a major management issue.

— AHT is evident when brain swelling is out of proportion to the size of the clot. This may be recognized on CT scan by finding "more shift than clot."

— Over several hours, it progresses to large areas of hypodensity on CT scan in the affected hemisphere.

— Is often associated with poor clinical outcome.

— The early parenchymal change accounts for much of the increased intracranial hypertension, which may persist after removing the clot.

— Other anatomical features of SDH in abusive head trauma include clot location and concurrent enlarged subarachnoid spaces, also called **benign external hydrocephalus**, which is not related to the injury itself but is common in infancy.

SDH FROM SHAKING

— Is often found near the midline in the interhemispheric space or perifalcine region.

— Posterior fossa SDH is also seen, often close to the tentorium.

— Subdural hemorrhage may be acute (hyperdense on CT scan), chronic (hypodense on CT scan), or mixed density.

1. Mixed-density SDH usually suggests serial bleeding from repeated episodes of abuse but may follow a single traumatic event.

2. Traumatic injury to the arachnoid membrane can mix CSF and subdural blood.[6]

CHRONIC SDH

— Is usually slightly hyperdense to CSF on CT scan but can be so hypodense as to mimic CSF density. Magnetic resonance imaging readily differentiates blood and CSF.

— Is termed **subdural hygroma** if CSF collection persists after the hematoma resolves.

— When ICP increases, shunting is needed (**Figure 4-4**). This situation is rare.

MANAGEMENT

— Surgery is predicated on the child's condition.

1. If awake and tolerating a small SDH, expectant management may be appropriate.

2. If comatose from diffuse brain injury with a tiny SDH, ICP monitoring may be appropriate.

3. If symptomatic for a large SDH, urgent evacuation of the hematoma is necessary.

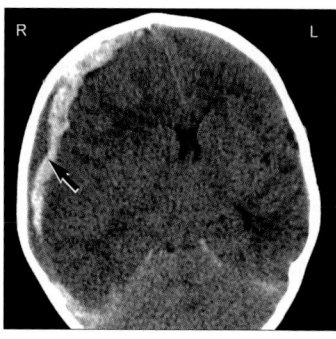

— The most common surgical options for acute hematomas are serial tapping, transfontanel drains, and/or craniotomy.

Figure 4-4. CT scan of 9-month-old boy found unresponsive. Mixed-density appearance of the subdural hematoma (arrow) found to contain both active bleeding and organized clot (hyperacute) bleeding.

1. Infants with an open fontanel:

    A. Obtain access to the subdural space percutaneously, assuming the fontanel is wide enough to avoid injury to the superior sagittal sinus with the needle and the hematoma is close to midline.

    B. Can perform tapping with a needle, which is then removed. Repeat as needed.

2. An alternative would be to access the subdural space using a standard intravenous catheter attached to a closed drainage system.

3. If the hematoma cannot be reached from the fontanel or the clot has a large, solid component, do a craniotomy.

    A. Make a large flap, taking care in opening the dura mater. When the brain is edematous in association with a thin clot, a widely opened dura mater can permit gross herniation of cerebral tissue, difficulties closing the wound, and further damage to the brain.

    B. An option is to do a craniotomy in the standard fashion but open the dura mater in a series of small slits, evacuating the hematoma in each area and closing each durotomy before opening the next.

    C. Perform postoperative ICP monitoring.

— After acute phase of management:

1. Close follow-up is necessary because of the risk of an enlarging, chronic hematoma. If this occurs, chronic macrocephaly can develop and the hematoma will not resolve spontaneously.

2. In this case, a shunt, with or without a low-pressure valve, is placed from the subdural space to the peritoneum, controlling the collection in the subdural space until brain growth allows brain volume to "catch up" to the size of the skull.

3. Once the hematoma has resolved and head growth has stabilized, consider removing the shunt if the family so desires. The shunt tube is a visible reminder of events surrounding the injury.[7,8]

OTHER SEVERE BRAIN INJURIES
— Various lesions may be present in a single case, but general management principles are the same.

— The comatose child is managed in the ICU setting with full hemodynamic monitoring.

1. ICP monitoring is performed with modifications to accommodate the thin skull.

2. A ventriculostomy or an intraparenchymal or subdural fiberoptic device is generally used.

3. Epidural pressure monitoring devices are inaccurate and not recommended.

4. The common assertion that a child with an open fontanel and open sutures cannot develop elevated ICP is not supported by data. This belief can result in undermanagement of a severely injured child, with untoward outcome.

5. The general goal is to maintain the infant in a normovolemic state with a cerebral perfusion pressure (CPP) of at least 40 to 50 mm Hg or ICP of less than 15 to 20 mm Hg.

6. Rising ICP or falling CPP indicates the need for repeated imaging, with surgery to remove expanding mass lesions.[9-11]

POSTTRAUMATIC HYDROCEPHALUS
— Is a late complication of severe closed head injury independent of mechanism.

— Occurs most often with intracranial hemorrhage related to injury, whether intraventricular, subarachnoid, or subdural.

— Standard ventriculoperitoneal shunting is used, though a lower closing pressure valve may be needed to address normal pressure hydrocephalus.

REFERENCES
1. Kruse JJ, Awasthi D. Skull-base trauma: neurosurgical perspective. *J Craniomaxillofac Trauma*. 1998;4:7-14.

2. Duke BJ, Mouchantat RA, Ketch LL, Winston KR. Transcranial migration of microfixation plates and screws. Case report. *Pediatr Neurosurg*. 1996;25:31-35.

3. McBride DQ, Murali R, Rovit RL. Depressed skull fractures. *Contemp Neurosurg*. 1988;10:1-6.

4. Choux M. Incidence, diagnosis and management of skull fractures. In: Raimondi AJ, Choux M, Di Rocco C, eds. *Head Injuries in the Newborn and Infant*. New York, NY: Springer-Verlag; 1986:163-182.

5. Piatt JH, Kernan JC. Intracranial hematomas. In: McLone DG, ed. *Pediatric Neurosurgery: Surgery of the Developing Nervous System*. 4th ed. Philadelphia, Pa: WB Saunders; 2001:634-645.

6. Vinchon M, Noizet O, DeFoort-Dhellemmes S, Soto-Ares G, Dhellemmes P. Infantile subdural hematomas due to traffic accidents. *Pediatr Neurosurg*. 2002;37:245-253.

7. Duhaime AC. Closed head injury without fractures. In: Albright AL, Pollack IF, Adelson PD, eds. *Principles and Practice of Pediatric Neurosurgery*. New York, NY: Thieme; 1999;799-811.

8. Duhaime AD, Partington MD. Overview and clinical presentation of inflicted head injury in infants. *Neurosurg Clin N Am*. 2002; 13:149-154.

9. Beaumont A, Marmarou A, Ward J. Intracranial hypertension mechanisms and management. In: McLone DG, ed. *Pediatric Neurosurgery: Surgery of the Developing Nervous System*. 4th ed. Philadelphia, Pa: WB Saunders; 2001:619-633.

10. Forbes ML, Kochanek PM, Adelson PD. Severe traumatic brain injury: critical care management. In: Albright AL, Pollack IF, Adelson PD, eds. *Principles and Practice of Pediatric Neurosurgery*. New York, NY: Thieme; 1999:861-878.

11. Stevenson KL, Adelson PD. Neurointensive care of the nonaccidentally injured child. *Neurosurg Clin N Am*. 2002;13:213-226.

Chapter 5

OPHTHALMOLOGY

Lori D. Frasier, MD, FAAP
Robert O. Hoffman, MD
Nick Mamalis, MD

EYE ANATOMY RELATED TO ABUSIVE HEAD TRAUMA

— The human eye is relatively protected by the bony orbit, eyelids, and conjunctiva.

— It is supported, cushioned, and moves along with muscles, motor nerves, fat, and connective tissue.

— Blood is supplied through various branches of the ophthalmic artery.

— Communication of neurologic impulses between the eye and the brain occurs via the optic nerve.

GLOBE (**Figures 5-1, 5-2,** and **5-3**)

— *Globe* is synonymous with *eyeball*.

— *Sclera.* Posterior ⅚ or outer layer of the eyeball; fibrous, opaque white covering.

— *Cornea.* Anterior ⅙ of the globe[1]; specialized connective tissue that remains clear.

— *Uvea.* Middle layer; includes the iris, ciliary body, and choroids.

1. *Iris.* Colored part of the eye; functions as a diaphragm with muscles that change pupil size in various lighting conditions.

2. *Ciliary body.* Wedge-shaped structure just posterior to the

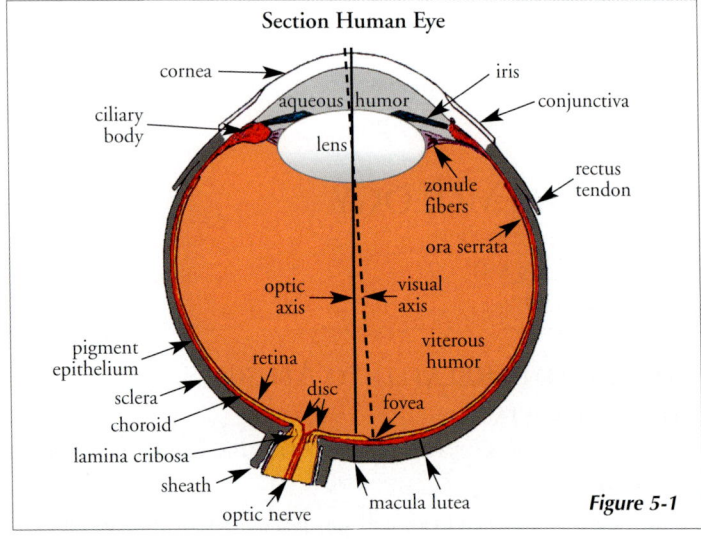

Figure 5-1. *Sagittal region of the globe. Reprinted with permission from Kolb, Fernandez, and Nelson.*[1]

Figure 5-2. *A sagittal section of a normal eye that has been removed and fixed in formalin, demonstrating the optic nerve (A), optic nerve head (B), an artifactual retinal fold (arrow C), the orra serrata at the anterior extent of the retina (arrow D), the cornea (arrow E), and the lens (arrow F). Both the lens and the cornea are opaque due to formalin fixation.*

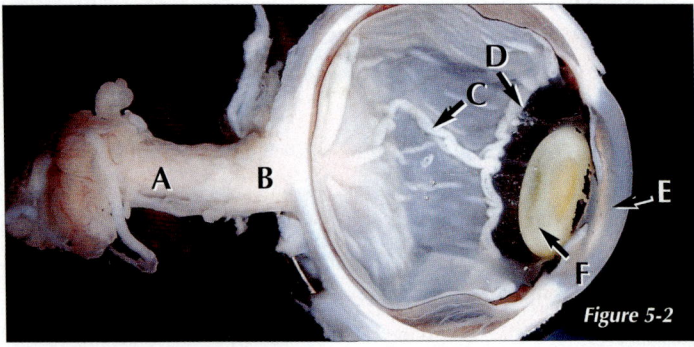

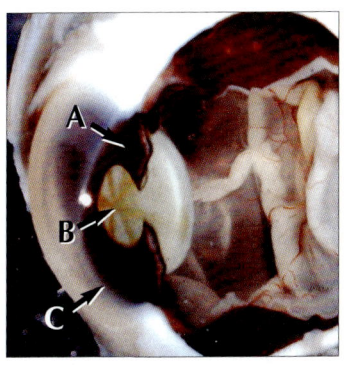

Figure 5-3. Normal anatomy of an eye that has been removed at autopsy, fixed in formalin, and cut in a parasagittal section. The iris (arrow A), lens (arrow B), and cornea (arrow C) are demonstrated. Note the retina. The folds and the brown, star-shaped change in the lens are artifacts of fixation in formalin.

peripheral iris; provides support to the lens and contains muscles that allow the lens to focus; where aqueous humor is produced.

3. ***Choroid.*** Vascular pigmented layer that helps decrease light scattering and provides blood supply to the outer retina, including photoreceptors.

— ***Inner layer.*** Retina and retinal pigment epithelium.

1. The neurosensory ***retina*** is a complex, multilayered structure[1] (**Figure 5-4**).

   A. Light energy is transformed into chemical and electrical signals, which are transmitted to the brain via the optic nerve.

   B. Visual information passes through the optic chiasm, where crossing of fibers allows each eye to send information to both sides of brain, passing through the optic tract, lateral geniculate, and optic radiation on its way to the visual cortex in the occipital lobe.

2. Photoreceptors are in the outermost layer of the retina.

   A. The 2 major types are rods and cones.

   B. ***Cones*** subserve fine discrimination and color perception.

   C. ***Rods*** permit sense of movement, peripheral vision, and dim light vision.

3. The ***retinal pigment epithelium:***

   A. Is just outside photoreceptors.

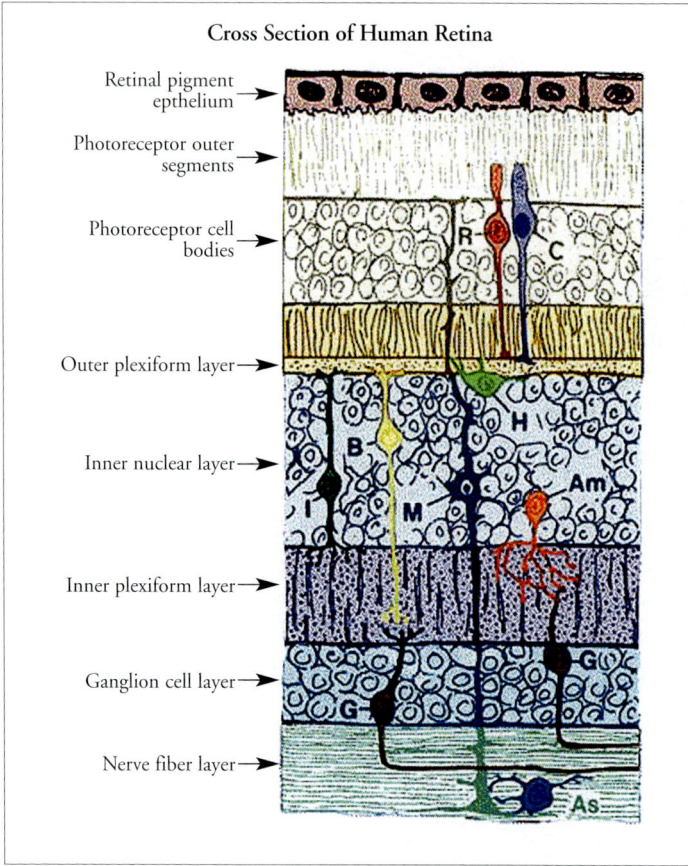

Cross Section of Human Retina

Retinal pigment epthelium →

Photoreceptor outer segments →

Photoreceptor cell bodies →

Outer plexiform layer →

Inner nuclear layer →

Inner plexiform layer →

Ganglion cell layer →

Nerve fiber layer →

Figure 5-4. *Cross section of human retina. Reprinted from Ogden,[2] with permission from Elsevier.*

    B. Provides nutrition and metabolic support to rods and cones.

    C. Is separated from the choroid by Bruch's membrane.

— Moving inward from the photoreceptors, alternating layers of cell bodies and their connections are found.

1. These permit specialized information processing from multiple rods and cones.

2. Axons of the innermost cell layer (ganglion cell layer) become the nerve fiber layer of the retina and join to leave the eye as the optic nerve.

— The *vitreous body* is the clear, gel-like substance in the posterior of the globe; composed mainly of water, hyaluronic acid, and collagen. Its consistency changes from relatively solid in infancy to more liquid with age.

— Attachments of the vitreous body to surrounding structures may be important in the pathophysiology of retinal hemorrhages (RHs) in abusive head trauma (AHT).

1. The *vitreous base* is an area where the vitreous body is firmly attached to the posterior ciliary body and anterior retina.

2. Attachments are also found between the vitreous body and the retina surrounding the optic nerve, over the macula and retinal vessels.

LENS
— The lens is an optically clear structure that helps focus light on the retina.

— *Zonules* are fibers that tether the lens to the ciliary body and help stabilize it. They allow the ciliary body to change shape in a controlled way so the eye can focus on near objects.

ROLE OF THE PEDIATRIC OPHTHALMOLOGIST
— Detect and carefully document RHs. This may require bedside consultation or an office examination.

— Document the quantity, location, and type of hemorrhages with drawings, photographs, or both as a member of the multidisciplinary team assessing the child.

— Perform a complete examination of visual behavior, pupils, external and anterior segments, and funduscopic findings to detect ophthalmic issues.

— Clinical care may require coordination among pediatric critical care specialists, neurosurgeons, child abuse specialists, and various ophthalmological subspecialists.

— Provide follow-up.

1. Monitor for resolution of RHs and potential vision-threatening problems.

2. Perform added testing (eg, electroretinogram to assess retinal function and the ***visual evoked potential test*** to assess optic nerve and central visual pathway function).

3. Address any treatable problems that require surgical intervention.

— Accurately convey ocular findings to other physicians caring for the child, the family, those deciding on placement of the child, law enforcement personnel, and various professionals involved in the legal system.

— Provide written documentation and participate in case conferences, depositions, or court testimony.

— Supply unbiased, factual information based on the best and most current evidence-based data available.

— Include acute findings and prognostic assessment based on subsequent testing and the most recent examination.

TOOLS

— Indirect ophthalmoscope (**Figure 5-5**):

1. Is used to obtain a thorough retinal examination and inspect the anterior segment and external tissues.

2. May require sedation and/or general anesthesia to obtain a detail-ed look at the retinal periphery.

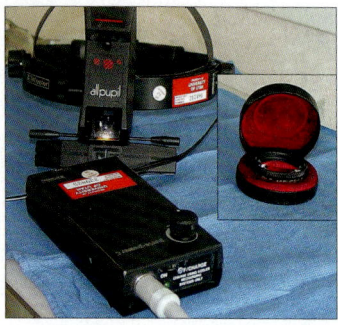

Figure 5-5. *The indirect ophthalmoscope, lens, and power source.*

3. Examination of the retina and periphery is difficult in awake, struggling children. It is often easier in the intensive care unit, when children are comatose or sedated.

— Lid speculum and scleral depressor allow better visualization of the periphery but use requires judgment regarding potential for patient harm (**Figure 5-6**).

— Detailed retinal drawings or digital fundus photographs (**Figure 5-7**) are often helpful additions to the medical record.

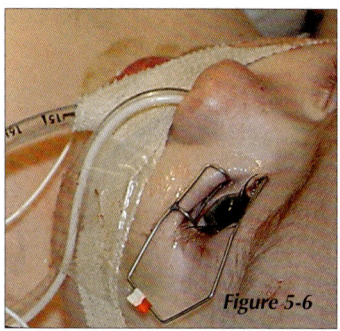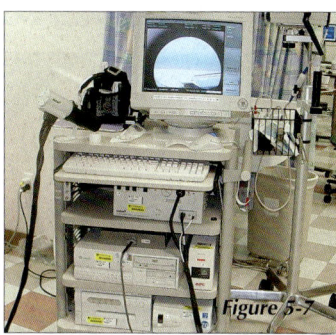

Figure 5-6

Figure 5-7

Figure 5-6. *The eyelid speculum may be used by the ophthalmologist for optimal exposure of the eye during examination with the RetCam or indirect ophthalmoscope.*

Figure 5-7. *RetCam digital imaging system including computer, monitor, light source, and printer.*

FINDINGS IN AHT

— A central ocular feature is retinal bleeding (**Figures 5-8-a** and **b**).

— Hemorrhages affect all retinal layers. Their appearance can help distinguish depth.

1. Preretinal hemorrhages:

    A. Lie between the retina and vitreous body.

    B. Often appear bullous (**Figure 5-8-b** and **Figure 5-9**).

    C. Boat shape reflects separation of blood components and settling of red blood cells by gravity when the patient is erect.

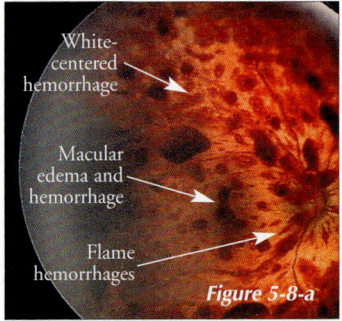

White-centered hemorrhage

Macular edema and hemorrhage

Flame hemorrhages

Figure 5-8-a

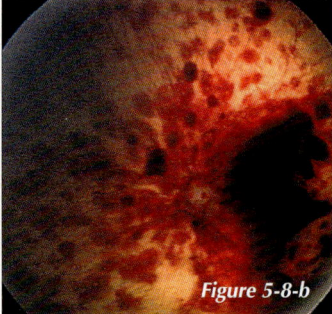

Figure 5-8-b

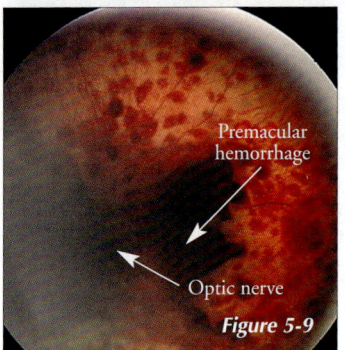

Premacular hemorrhage

Optic nerve

Figure 5-9

Figure 5-8-a. RetCam image of fundus oculus dexter with flame and white-centered hemorrhages, which are typical of SBS.

Figure 5-8-b. RetCam image of fundus oculus sinister with flame and white-centered hemorrhages.

Figure 5-9. RetCam image with premacular hemorrhage.

2. Superficial RHs:

    A. Lie between the retina and internal limiting membrane.

    B. Often have circular, raised appearance.

3. Slightly deeper hemorrhages in the nerve fiber layer are flame-shaped.

4. Still deeper RHs have a dot or blot appearance.

5. Very deep or subretinal hemorrhages:

    A. Have a darker appearance.

    B. Lie beneath retinal blood vessels.

— The location and extent of hemorrhages are also important to note.

— Other significant ocular findings include retinal folds (**Figure 5-10** and **Figure 5-11**) or retinoschisis, hemorrhage in the vitreous body, choroid, optic nerve sheath[3,4] (**Figure 5-12**), and sclera surrounding the optic nerve.[5]

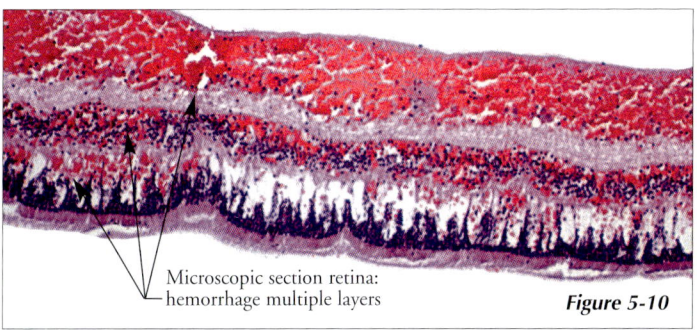

Microscopic section retina: hemorrhage multiple layers

Figure 5-10

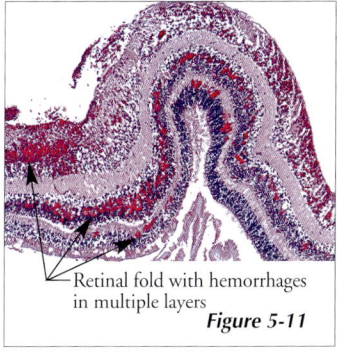

Retinal fold with hemorrhages in multiple layers

Figure 5-11

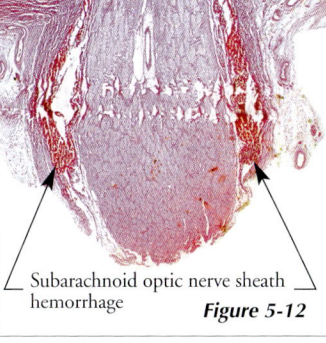

Subarachnoid optic nerve sheath hemorrhage

Figure 5-12

Figure 5-10. *Hemorrhage in multiple layers. (Photograph courtesy of Nick Mamalis, MD.)*

Figure 5-11. *Retinal fold with hemorrhages in multiple layers. (Photograph courtesy of Nick Mamalis, MD.)*

Figure 5-12. *Illustration of subarachnoid optic nerve sheath hemorrhage. (Photograph courtesy of Nick Mamalis, MD.)*

1. Retinal folds indicate severe acceleration-deceleration injury.[6-8]

2. Retinoschisis:

    A. Involves anatomical and functional abnormalities, including decreased visual acuity. Electroretinogram results are abnormal.

    B. Requires thorough medical and investigative process to determine the cause.

    C. No current clinical or scientific information suggests that retinoschisis involving decreased visual acuity and abnormal electroretinogram results occurs in any circumstance other than severe trauma.[9]

3. Vitreous hemorrhage:

    A. Is a negative prognostic indicator. Decreased vision is expected with prolonged interference with formed visual input.[10]

    B. Vitreous and choroidal hemorrhage may indicate more serious injury.[11,12]

— Possible mechanisms of injury with shaken baby syndrome (SBS) include:

1. Direct extension of intracranial blood.

2. Transmitted increased venous pressure with rupture of vessels.

3. Local rupture of vessels from differential movement of intraocular and intraorbital tissues associated with acceleration-deceleration forces.

4. *Terson syndrome* is intraocular bleeding associated with subarachnoid hemorrhage.

5. Perimacular retinal folds and retinoschisis provide evidence for acceleration and deceleration of tissues.[6,13]

DIFFERENTIAL DIAGNOSIS

— It is essential to identify patients for whom the diagnosis of child abuse is not appropriate.[14,15]

— There are no absolutely pathognomonic ocular findings.[15-18]

— The appropriate diagnosis often depends on the disparity between the injuries observed and the suggested mechanism according to the caregiver's history.[19]

— A history of minimal accidental head trauma is common.

— In the absence of severe head trauma or central nervous system disease, ocular findings, including retinal, peripheral retinal, intrascleral, and optic nerve sheath hemorrhages, are diagnostic of child abuse.

— Hydrocephalus can cause RHs with increased intracranial pressure, but these are usually limited to the peripapillary retinal area.

— Various hematological abnormalities (leukemias, aplastic anemia, von Willebrand disease, vitamin K deficiency, disseminated intravascular coagulation, Henoch-Schonlein purpura, and protein S or C deficiency) are associated with RHs.[20-23] Affected patients are identifiable based on clinical features, abnormal complete blood cell count, or aberrant coagulation studies.

— Glutaricaciduria type I is associated with intraretinal hemorrhages.

1. Hemorrhages are located near the vascular arcade and are seen when the patient is encephalopathic.

2. Vitreous hemorrhage is rare in galactosemia with coagulopathy.[24]

3. Typical history and clinical features (as well as serological testing) permit diagnosis of hemorrhages.

— Other disorders associated with RHs in infancy are retinopathy of prematurity (ROP),[25] meningococcal meningitis,[20] recent intraocular surgery,[26] and severe hypertension.[20]

1. Distinguish based on history or other clinical features.

2. It is possible that the child has one of these conditions and has been abused.

— Unilateral hemorrhages occur in up to 50% of AHT cases.[4,27-29]

— There is a low incidence of RHs after cardiopulmonary resuscitation.

— Most children suspected of SBS have evidence of blunt head trauma at autopsy.[30,31]

— RHs are more frequent in SBS victims than in those with blunt trauma alone.[32]

— Potentially fragile vessels may relate to ROP.

1. Mild ROP causes vitreous hemorrhages at a threshold of trauma that would not cause bleeding from more mature vessels.

2. Though infants with ROP can be victims of AHT, they can have retinal and vitreous hemorrhages without AHT, so use caution in interpreting findings.

3. In infants with significant ROP and suspected AHT, consultation with an ophthalmologist knowledgeable and skilled in evaluating both disorders is recommended.

— Subdural hematoma and intraocular bleeding in SBS may be caused by severe hypoxia, brain edema, and increased central venous pressure, which can occur without significant impact or force.[33]

— Hypoxic injury may cause some SBS changes, but not all.

PATHOLOGY

— Pathologic examination is required to reveal findings such as optic nerve sheath and periopticointrascleral hemorrhages (**Figures 5-13-a, b, and c**).[3,5,8,11,31]

— Perimacular folds can be found clinically[6] and confirmed by histopathological report.

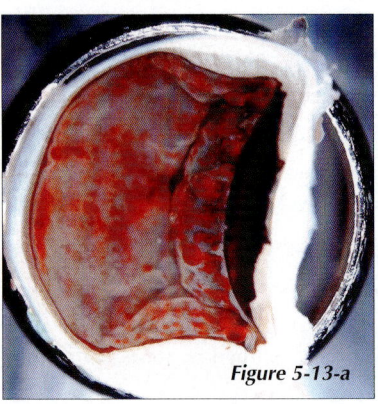

Figure 5-13-a. *Sagittal section of an eye removed at autopsy from a child who died from AHT. The red coloration of the retina is due to extensive retinal hemorrhage extending from the posterior pole to the ora serrata.*

Figure 5-13-a

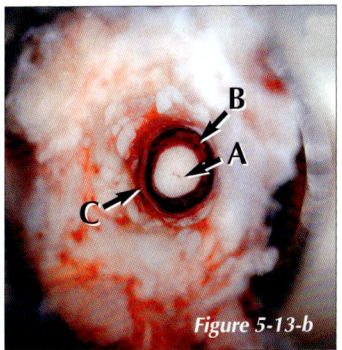
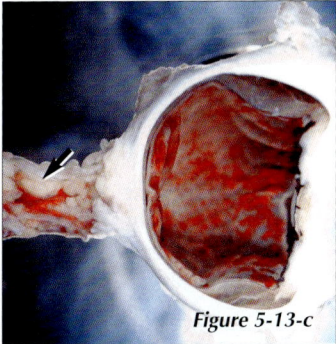

Figure 5-13-b. *Optic nerve (arrow A) in cross section with optic nerve sheath hemorrhages (arrows B and C).*

Figure 5-13-c. *Cross section of the optic nerve (arrow) from an eye that has been fixed in formalin, demonstrating hemor-rhage between optic nerve sheath and optic nerve.*

REFERENCES

1. Kolb H, Fernandez E, Nelson R. Webvision Web site. January 2005. Available at: http://webvision.med.utah.edu. Accessed May 18, 2005.

2 Ogden TE. *Retina: Basic Science and Inherited Retinal Disease.* St. Louis, Mo: Mosby; 1989.

3. Lambert SR, Johnson TE, Hoyt CS. Optic nerve sheath and retinal hemorrhages associated with the shaken baby syndrome. *Arch Ophthalmol.* 1986;104:1509-1512.

4. Budenz DL, Farber MG, Mirchandani HG, Park H, Rorke LB. Ocular and optic nerve hemorrhages in abused infants with intra-cranial injuries. *Ophthalmology.* 1994;101:559-565.

5. Lin KC, Glasgow BJ. Bilateral periopticointrascleral hemorrhages associated with traumatic child abuse. *Am J Ophthalmol.* 1999; 127:473-475.

6. Gaynon MW, Koh K, Marmor MF, Frankel LR. Retinal folds in the shaken baby syndrome. *Am J Ophthalmol.* 1988;106:423-425.

7. Massicotte SJ, Folberg R, Torczynski E, Gilliland MG, Luckenbach MW. Vitreoretinal traction and perimacular retinal folds in the eyes of deliberately traumatized children. *Ophthalmology.* 1991;98:1124-1127.

8. Munger CE, Peiffer RL, Bouldin TW, Kylstra JA, Thompson RL. Ocular and associated neuropathologic observations in suspected whiplash shaken infant syndrome. A retrospective study of 12 cases. *Am J Forensic Med Pathol.* 1993;14:193-200.

9. Lantz PE, Sinal SH, Stanton CA, Weaver RG Jr. Perimacular retinal folds from childhood head trauma. *BMJ.* 2004;328:754-756.

10. Matthews GP, Das A. Dense vitreous hemorrhages predict poor visual and neurological prognosis in infants with shaken baby syndrome. *J Pediatr Ophthalmol Strabismus.* 1996;33:260-265.

11. Green MA, Lieberman G, Milroy CM, Parsons MA. Ocular and cerebral trauma in non-accidental injury in infancy: underlying mechanisms and implications for paediatric practice. *Br J Ophthalmol.* 1996;80:282-287.

12. Wilkinson WS, Han DP, Rappley MD, Owings CL. Retinal hemorrhage predicts neurologic injury in the shaken baby syn-drome. *Arch Ophthalmol.* 1989;107:1472-1474.

13. Greenwald MJ, Weiss A, Oesterle CS, Friendly DS. Traumatic retinoschisis in battered babies. *Ophthalmology.* 1986;93:618-625.

14. Kirschner RH, Stein RJ. The mistaken diagnosis of child abuse. A form of medical abuse? *Am J Dis Child.* 1985;139:873-875.

15. Weissgold DJ, Budenz DL, Hood I, Rorke LB. Ruptured vascular malformation masquerading as battered/shaken baby syndrome: a nearly tragic mistake. *Surv Ophthalmol.* 1995;38:509-512.

16. Gilkes MJ, Mann TP. Fundi of battered babies. *Lancet.* 1967;2: 468.

17. Kessler DB, Siegel-Stein F. Retinal hemorrhage, meningitis, and child abuse. *NY State J Med.* 1984;84:59-60.

18. Tongue AC. The ophthalmologist's role in diagnosing child abuse. *Ophthalmology*. 1991;93:1009-1010.

19. Lancon JA, Haines DE, Parent AD. Anatomy of the shaken baby syndrome. *Anat Rec*. 1998;253:13-18.

20. The Ophthalmology Child Abuse Working Party. Child abuse and the eye. *Eye*. 1999;13(pt 1):3-10.

21. Levin AV. Retinal hemorrhages and child abuse. In: David TJ, ed. *Recent Advances in Paediatrics*. Vol 18. London, England: Churchill Livingstone; 2000:151-219.

22. Mansour AM, Salti HI, Han DP, et al. Ocular findings in aplastic anemia. *Ophthalmologica*. 2000;214:399-402.

23. Shiono T, Abe S, Watabe T, et al. Vitreous, retinal and subretinal hemorrhages associated with von Willebrand's syndrome. *Graefes Arch Clin Exp Ophthalmol*. 1992;230:496-497.

24. Levy HL, Brown AE, Williams SE, de Juan E. Vitreous hemorrhage as an ophthalmic complication of galactosemia. *J Pediatr*. 1996;129:922-925.

25. Kwok AK, So AK, Lam SW, Ng JS, Fok TF, Lam DS. Can vitreous hemorrhage indicate non-accidental injury if mild retinopathy of prematurity is present? *Eye*. 2000;14(pt 5):812-813.

26. Christiansen S, Munoz M, Capo H. Retinal hemorrhage following lensectomy and vitrectomy in children. *J Pediatr Ophthalmol Strabismus*. 1993;30:24-27.

27. Levin AV. Ocular manifestations of child abuse. *Ophthalmol Clin N Am*. 1990;3:249-264.

28. Betz P, Puschel K, Miltner E, Lignitz E, Eisenmenger W. Morphometical analysis of retinal hemorrhages in the shaken baby syndrome. *Forensic Sci Int*. 1996;78:71-80.

29. American Academy of Pediatrics: Committee on Child Abuse and Neglect. Shaken baby syndrome: rotational cranial injuries—technical report. *Pediatrics*. 2001;108:206-210.

30. Duhaime AC, Gennarelli TA, Thibault LE, Bruce DA, Margulies SS, Wiser R. The shaken baby syndrome. A clinical, pathological, and biomechanical study. *J Neurosurg.* 1987;66:409-415.

31. Elner SG, Elner VM, Arnall M, Albert DM. Ocular and associated systemic findings in suspected child abuse. A necropsy study. *Arch Ophthalmol.* 1990;108:1094-1101.

32. Gilliland MG, Folberg R. Shaken babies: some have no impact injuries. *J Forensic Sci.* 1996;411:114-116.

33. Geddes JF, Tasker RC, Hackshaw AK, et al. Dural haemorrhage in non-traumatic infant deaths: does it explain the bleeding in "shaken baby syndrome"? *Neuropathol Appl Neurobiol.* 2003;29:14-22.

Chapter

Associated Injuries

Randell Alexander, MD, PhD, FAAP

Scott A. Benton, MD, FAAP

Gail V. Benton, DDS

Bradford W. Betz, MD, MS

Lori D. Frasier, MD, FAAP

Robert N. Parrish, JD

Vincent J. Palusci, MD, MS

David A. Start, MD

— Any abusive injury can coexist with abusive head trauma (AHT) (**Table 6-1**).

— AHT caused by shaking can accompany injuries elsewhere that can significantly affect care. Children may survive AHT but die of the other injuries.

— Assume that all body parts are injured until proved otherwise.

— **Table 6-2** lists medical studies used to screen for associated injuries in suspected AHT. Many can be done simultaneously with studies that are conducted if AHT is the only condition being considered.

Review of Possible Injuries

Knowing the context in which the child is abused helps in understanding the circumstances contributing to the abuse as well as the range of risks faced.

Abdominal Trauma

— Is difficult to detect because external skin injuries are uncommon[1,2] (**Figure 6-1**).

Table 6-1. Possible Additional Injuries Observed in Children With SBS

OTHER HEAD INJURIES

— Bruises

— Fractures (eg, skull, orbital, nasal, or jaw fractures)

— Eye trauma (eg, hyphema or traumatic retinal detachments)

— Dental injuries (eg, teeth or frenulum)

NECK INJURIES

— Petechiae to the head and/or neck, possibly indicating strangulation

— Blood vessel damage, possibly from squeezing

— Tracheal injury

— Soft tissue injuries to the muscles or around the spinal cord

THORAX INJURIES

— Cardiac contusions and comotio cordis

— Hemothorax, chylothorax

— Pleural and lung injuries

ABDOMINAL INJURIES

— Solid organ injuries (eg, pancreas, liver, kidneys, or spleen)

— Hollow organ injuries (eg, intestines or stomach)

— Other injuries (eg, mesentery, bladder, or uterus)

GENITAL INJURIES

— Sexual or physical abuse injuries

BONE INJURIES

— Rib fractures

— Other fractures or injuries

SKIN INJURIES

— Bruises

— Burns

— Abrasions

(continued)

Table 6-1. *(continued)*

GROWTH PARAMETER PROBLEMS
— Failure to thrive

OTHER ISSUES
— Evidence of exposure to illegal drugs
— Hemoglobinuria, myoglobinuria

Table 6-2. Medical Studies in Cases of Suspected AHT

RECOMMENDED STUDIES

Related to Head Trauma
— Computed tomography (CT) scan of the head
— Magnetic resonance imaging (MRI) of the head
— Ophthalmological examination

Related to Injuries Other Than Head Trauma
— Skeletal survey for any child with AHT (not only for children younger than 2 years, which is the guideline for other forms of physical abuse); possible bone scan or repeated skeletal survey 2 weeks later to detect otherwise occult fractures
— Skin examination
— Genital examination (by a person trained in the procedure); follow-up forensic genital examination if any questions arise
— Growth parameter assessment (ie, to detect failure to thrive)

LABORATORY STUDIES
— Liver and pancreatic enzyme assessments
— Urinalysis for myoglobin and hemoglobin levels; urinalysis for presence of illegal drugs (eg, for cocaine or methamphetamine), indicating that it has been smoked in the child's presence—a finding that should be considered a form of abuse
— Complete blood count (CBC), prothrombin time (PT), partial thrombo-plastin time (PTT), platelets

(continued)

Table 6-2. *(continued)*

OPTIONAL STUDIES (DEPENDING ON SITUATION)

— CT scan of thorax and abdomen, which can easily be done as continuation of head CT scan; it only takes several seconds more with today's technology

— Dentistry consultation (a procedure that is often overlooked)

— Urinalysis (organic acids and metabolic studies)

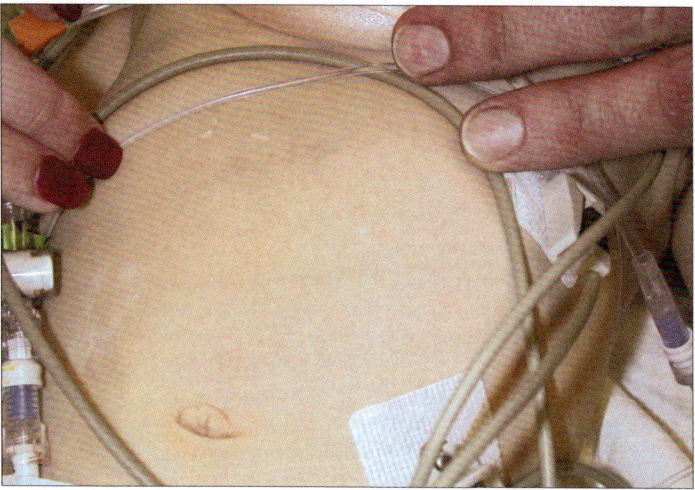

Figure 6-1. *Faint abdominal bruising to the abdomen and the lower costal margin.*

— Usually leads to internal bleeding, infection, or both.

— The extent of the symptoms is a developing phenomenon that occurs as bleeding or infection progresses.

— Symptoms may develop late or care may be delayed by the person who abused the child.

— Symptoms of abdominal trauma can be confused with concurrent head trauma.

— Physical examination alone is a poor, unreliable predictor of abdominal injury.

SEXUAL ABUSE

— No substantive literature documents the coexistence of sexual abuse and AHT.

1. Typical ages at which each type of abuse occurs differ.

    A. AHT caused by shaking is most common in children younger than 1 year.

    B. Sexual abuse is more common in older children.

2. Dynamics of each type of abuse:

    A. AHT is frequently the result of impulsive actions caused by anger.

    B. Sexual abuse is most commonly the result of sexual desire satisfied in a planned process or undertaken in a moment of opportunity.

— Consider sexual abuse in all children who suffer abusive injuries.

— Sexual abuse and physical abuse are more likely to occur together when the abuser uses drugs or alcohol, both of which lower inhibitory impulses (**Figure 6-2**).

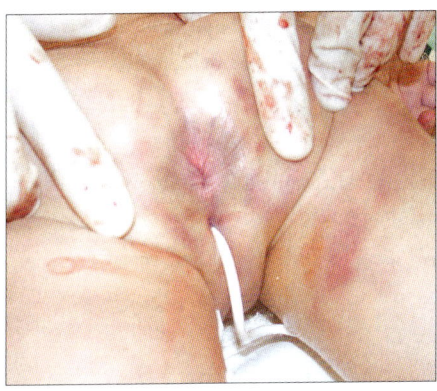

Figure 6-2. *Perianal bruising indicating sexual assault, which may have precipitated the perpetrator striking the child's head against a hard surface, resulting in the brain and skull injuries.*

— Men are more likely than women to be sexually abusive and to cause physical abuse injuries, including shaken baby syndrome (SBS).[3,4]

Drug Exposure

— Children are rarely tested for drugs as part of the physical examination for child abuse.

— Benzoylecgonine:

1. Is the primary metabolite of cocaine and can be detected in urine.

2. About 4% of the urine of newborns and older children in the United States tested for benzoylecgonine shows evidence of cocaine exposure.[5-8] Urine levels are comparable regardless of exposure method.

   A. Newborns receive cocaine from the mother via the umbilical cord before birth.

   B. Older children can be exposed through passive inhalation of cocaine smoke (crack) in the environment.

— Methamphetamine and marijuana:

1. Are common smokable drugs that leave detectable urine levels in children.

2. Exposure of a child to illegal substances that leads to a positive drug test is considered a form of child abuse in some states.

3. May be a factor when considering the child's placement.

Bone Injuries

— Forces exerted on the body may cause skeletal injuries.

— The child may be hit directly; have limbs twisted, grabbed, or pulled; or suffer other injuries to the bones.

— May also signify previous assaults independent of specific abusive injuries.

— Skull fractures:

1. Are caused by direct impact to the head (**Figures 6-3-a** and **b**).

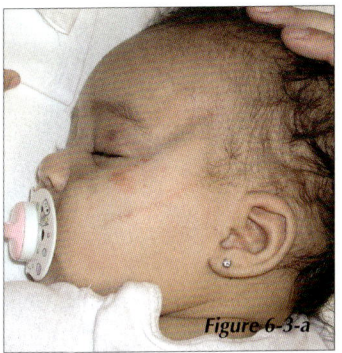
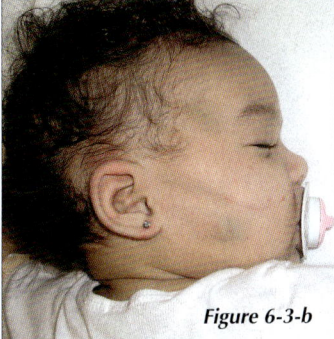

Figures 6-3-a and **b.** *Slap marks to both sides of a 5-month-old girl's face. She was found to have right posterior cerebral and interhemispheric subdural hematomas with layering over the tentorium.*

2. The presence of more diffuse brain damage than expected from purely focal impacts and substantial retinal hemorrhages demonstrates that shaking was significant, but that it was not the only factor in these injuries.

— Neck injuries:

1. It is a misconception that the neck must be injured in shaking. This misconception is based on adult whiplash injuries with trauma.

2. Neck injuries are very rare in children with SBS. They are found in only 2% to 5% of all children who die.[9]

3. Evidence of soft tissue injury and damage around the spinal cord can be seen at autopsy of children who have neck injuries and die from SBS.

4. Substantial spinal cord injury is even less common and may suggest direct trauma to the neck.

5. Bone injuries caused by shaking alone are either exceptionally rare or do not occur.[10]

— Injury to long bones of arms and legs:

1. It has been suggested that limbs may flail sufficiently during shaking to cause stress on the ends of the long bones of the arms and legs,[11] producing metaphyseal fractures.

2. The original descriptions of SBS included fractured arms and legs; however, such fractures are not necessary to diagnose AHT and are not part of the specific definition of SBS.

3. Metaphyseal injuries can also result when children's arms or legs are twisted and pulled during physical abuse that does not produce injuries related to SBS (**Figures 6-4-a** and **b**).

— Rib fractures:

1. Are caused by a direct impact with concentrated force, such as kicking or punching; occur when an adult vigorously squeezes a

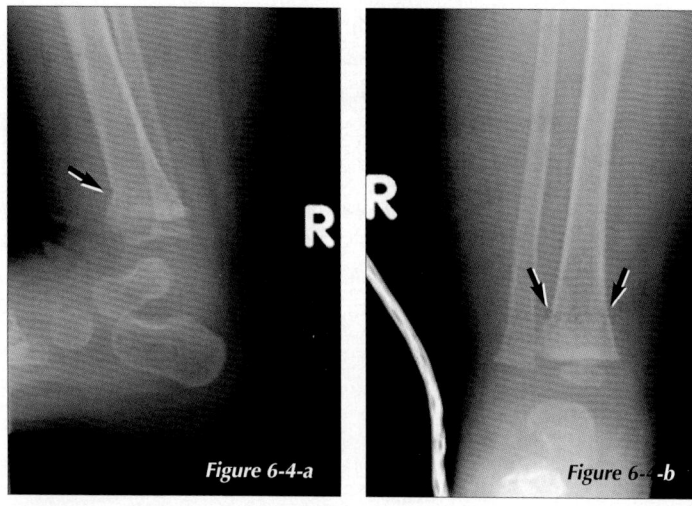

Figure 6-4-a. Lateral view of tibia and fibula of 9-month-old girl. The tibial fracture (arrow) is most apparent as a cortical defect.

Figure 6-4-b. Anteroposterior view of the tibia and fibula showing the tibial fracture (arrows).

child's chest or when a child is held around the torso during abusive acts such as shaking. The gripping of the rib cage is reinforced by the forces of the chest moving back and forth, creating pressure.

2. Forces spread out over a broad surface area are normally insufficient to cause children's flexible ribs to break.

3. Are not seen in infants and very young children who fall from considerable heights.

4. Posterior rib fractures can occur during bimanual compression and levering at the costotransverse process articulations.[12]

5. Are not typically detected during a physical examination and tend to appear on chest radiographs (**Figure 6-5**).

6. External bruising over a rib fracture is rare. Healing rib fractures rarely have a history of chest bruising.

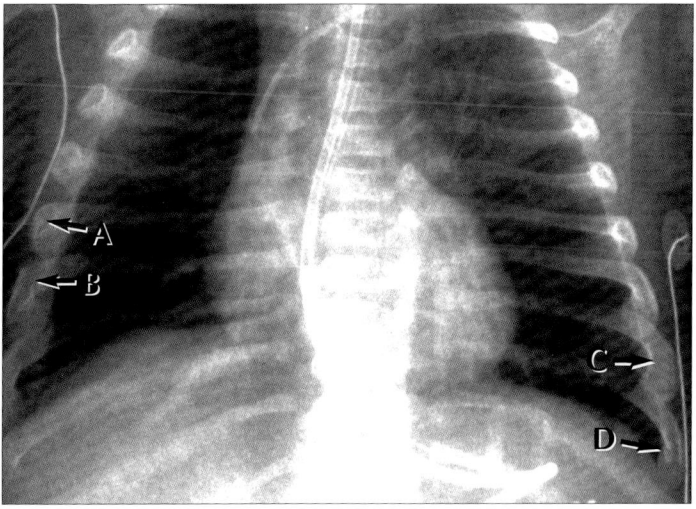

Figure 6-5. *AP chest radiograph of 6-week-old girl with seizures and multiple injuries demonstrating healing fractures of the right lateral sixth and seventh ribs (arrows A and B) and the left lateral seventh and eighth ribs (arrows C and D).*

— Approximately 50% of children with AHT caused by shaking with impact have evidence of some form of head impact (ie, skull fractures).[13]

— Skin injuries (patterns):

1. Slap marks (**Figures 6-6-a** and **b**)

2. Burns (**Figures 6-7-a, b, c,** and **d**)

3. Bites (**Figures 6-8-a** and **b**)

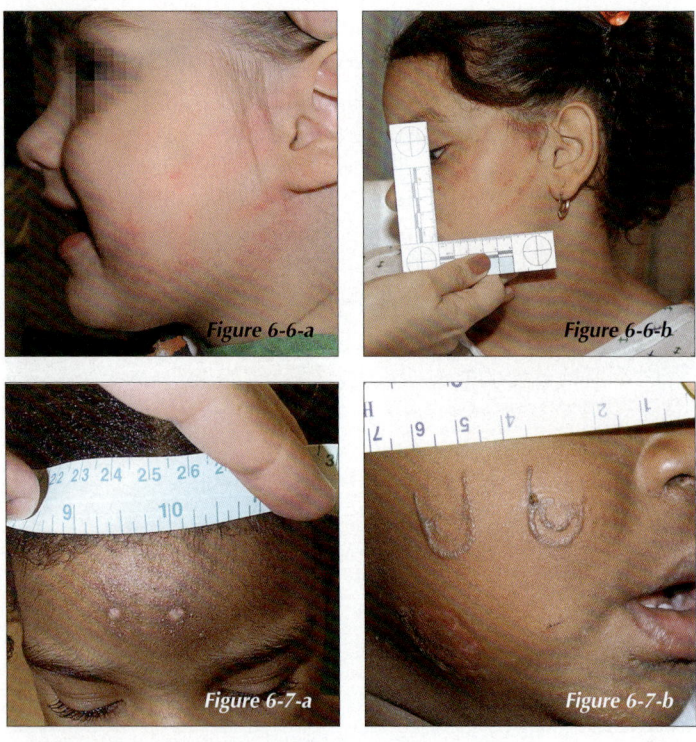

Figure 6-6-a

Figure 6-6-b

Figure 6-7-a

Figure 6-7-b

Figures 6-6-a and **b.** *Slap marks on the cheek.*

Figures 6-7-a to **d.** *Contact burns on the face.*

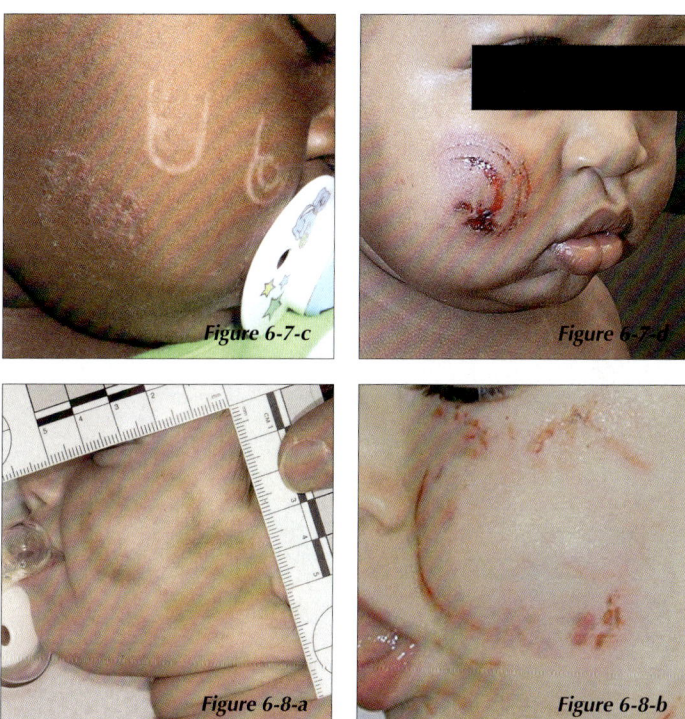

Figures 6-8-a and **b.** Human bite marks on the cheeks of infants.

— Oral injuries:

1. Lips (**Figure 6-9**)

2. Teeth (**Figures 6-10-a** and **b**)

— Eyes (**Figures 6-11-a** and **b; 6-12**)

Failure to Thrive

— Neglect is defined as chronic failure to attend to a child's needs. It is not an impulsive act.

— Neglectful adults rarely know that what they are doing is wrong.

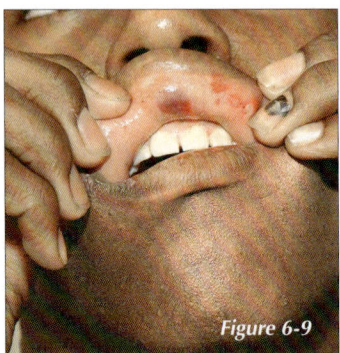

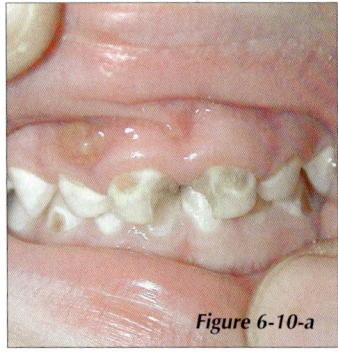

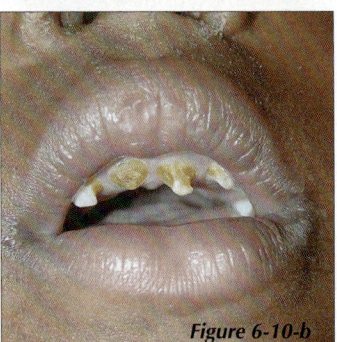

Figure 6-9. Lip injury caused by maltreatment.

Figures 6-10-a and **b.** Dental caries caused by neglect.

Figures 6-11-a and **b.** Hematoma to the mid forehead of 3-year-old child. Images document the injury the day of (a) and 2 days subsequent to the fall causing the injury (b).

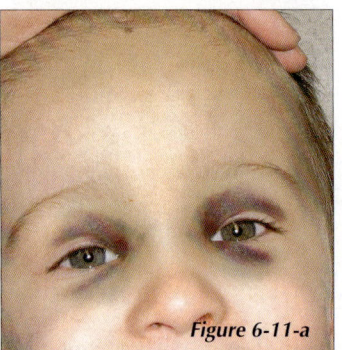

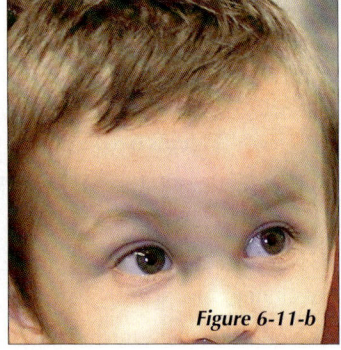

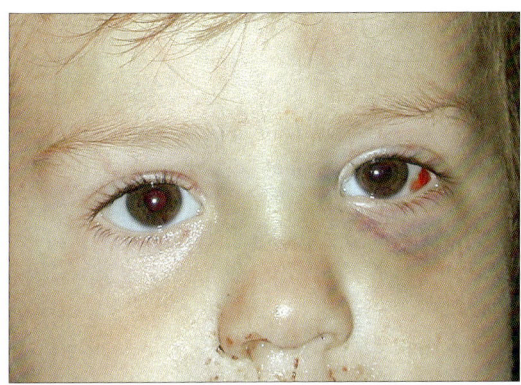

Figure 6-12. *Blunt trauma to the eyes.*

— Neglect is the most commonly reported form of child abuse in the United States.

— It can be difficult to understand the severity of the neglect when confronted with the obvious injuries of physical abuse.

— Long-term outcomes can be serious or fatal.

— Carefully examine all data in the child's life to correctly characterize the overall abusive environment.

INJURIES TO OTHERS
— The siblings of an abused child can also be victims of abuse.

— Twins and other children of multiple births are at higher risk of concurrent abuse than other types of siblings.[14]

— Examine an apparently healthy child (physical examination, MRI of the head, skeletal survey, possible retinal examination) if the twin has been abused.

— Intimate partner violence may also be an issue; question caregivers carefully.

REFERENCES
1. Huyer D. Abdominal injuries in child abuse. *APSAC Advisor.* 1994;7:5-9.

2. Ledbetter DJ, Hatch EI Jr, Feldman KW, Fligner CL, Tapper D. Diagnostic and surgical implications of child abuse. *Arch Surg*. 1988;123:1101-1105.

3. Starling SP, Holden JR. Perpetrators of abusive head trauma: a comparison of two geographic populations. *South Med J*. 2000; 93:463-465.

4. US Advisory Board on Child Abuse and Neglect. *A Nation's Shame: Fatal Child Abuse and Neglect in the United States*. Washington, DC: US Dept of Health & Human Services; 1995.

5. Heidemann SM, Goetting MG. Passive inhalation of cocaine by infants. *Henry Ford Hosp Med J*. 1990;38:252-254.

6. Mirchandani HG, Mirchandani IH, Hellman F, English-Rider R, Rosen S, Laposata EA. Passive inhalation of free-base cocaine ("crack") smoke by infants. *Arch Pathol Lab Med*. 1991;115:494-498.

7. Rosenberg NM, Meert KL, Knazik SR, Yee H, Kauffman RE. Occult cocaine exposure in children. *Am J Dis Child*. 1991;145: 1430-1432.

8. Shannon M, Lacouture PB, Roa J, Woolf A. Cocaine exposure among children seen at a pediatric hospital. *Pediatrics*. 1989;83: 337-342.

9. Alexander R, Levitt C, Smith W. Abusive head trauma. In: Reece R, Ludwig W, eds. *Child Abuse: Medical Diagnosis and Management*. Philadelphia, Pa: Lippincott Williams & Wilkins; 2001: 47-80.

10. Feldman KW, Weinberger E, Milstein JM, Fligner CL. Cervical spine MRI in abused infants. *Child Abuse Negl*. 1997;21:199-205.

11. Kleinman PK. Diagnostic imaging in infant abuse. *AJR Am J Roentgenol*. 1990;155:703-712.

12. Kleinman PK, Schlesinger AE. Mechanical factors associated with posterior rib fractures: laboratory and case studies. *Pediatr Radiol*. 1997;27:87-91.

13. Alexander R, Sato Y, Smith W, Bennett T. Incidence of impact trauma with cranial injuries ascribed to shaking. *Am J Dis Child*. 1990;144:724-726.

14. Becker JC, Liersch R, Tautz C, Schlueter B, Andler W. Shaken baby syndrome: report on four pairs of twins. *Child Abuse Negl*. 1998;22:931-937.

Medical Disorders That Mimic Abusive Head Trauma

Lori D. Frasier, MD, FAAP
Andrew P. Sirotnak, MD

This chapter lists various conditions that may be considered in assessing a child for abusive head injury; it is not intended to be comprehensive.

Prenatal-, Perinatal-, and Pregnancy-Related Conditions

— *Intrauterine trauma.* History is unreliable in cases in which domestic violence is a factor. Differentiate by history and physical examination.

— *Domestic violence assault.* Differentiate by history, which may be unreliable.

— *Intrauterine isoimmune thrombocytopenia purpura.*[1] A rare condition in which maternal antibodies destroy fetal platelets. Differentiate by history and laboratory tests.

— *Maternal preeclampsia.* Rare; differentiate by history, physical examination, and laboratory tests.

— *Idiopathic intrauterine subdural hemorrhage (SDH).* Differentiate by history and radiology.

— *Postnatal cerebral infarction.* Differentiate by radiology.

— *Prenatal abdominal massage (urut).*[2] A cultural practice of Pacific Islanders. Differentiate by history, physical examination, and radiology.

Birth Trauma

— *Forceps delivery.*[3] Although rare, scalp trauma is often obvious. Differentiate by history and physical examination.

— *Vacuum extraction.*[4] May cause tentorial hemorrhage and potential significant injury. Differentiate by history and physical examination.

— *Breech delivery.*[3,5] Associated with a higher incidence of SDH. Differentiate by history and physical examination.

— *Ischemic stroke.*[6] Affects the vertebral, middle, and posterior cerebral arteries as a complication of direct trauma or temporal-herniation–induced compression. Differentiate by history, physical examination, and radiology.

Congenital Malformations

— *Intracranial arteriovenous malformations (AVMs).*[7,8] Cause congestive heart failure and cranial bruit in neonates and sudden severe headaches and increased intracranial pressure (ICP) in older children. Differentiate by radiology.

— *Cerebral aneurysm.*[9,10] Rupture usually causes subarachnoid hemorrhages (SAHs). Differentiate by radiology.

— *Osler-Weber-Rendu syndrome.*[11,12] A rare hereditary condition of AVM and aneurysm. Differentiate by history and radiology.

— *Arachnoid cysts.*[13] Ruptured vessels surrounding cysts produce SDH (**Figure 7-1**). Differentiate by radiology.

— *Congenital hydrocephalus.*[14] A manifestation of fetal SDH. Differentiate by history, physical examination, and radiology.

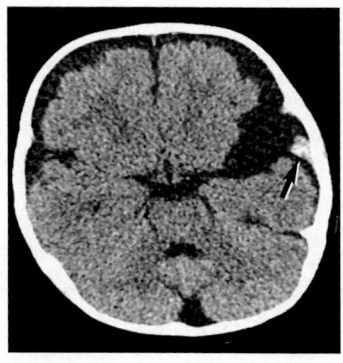

Figure 7-1. *Noncontrast computed tomography (CT) scan of 9-month-old boy showing left temporal fossa arachnoid cyst with an acute hemorrhage (arrow) and mass effect on the underlying brain.*

— *Encephalocele and meningocele.*[15,16] Congenital defects of the skull and brain in which bleeding can occur. Differentiate by history, physical examination, and radiology.

— *Acquired syringomyelia.* Differentiate by history, physical examination, and radiology.

— *Spontaneous rupture of the cerebral artery.* Reported only in adults.

— *Spontaneous spinal epidural hematoma.*[17] Rare in infants and children. Differentiate by physical examination and radiology.

— *Spontaneous SAHs.*[18] Not found as isolated events in children.

— *Spontaneous SDH.* Reported only in adults.

— *Superior sagittal sinus thrombosis.*[19-22] Nearly always related to an underlying or preexisting condition. Differentiate by history, radiology, and laboratory tests.

MEDICAL CONDITIONS LINKED TO SUPERIOR SAGITTAL SINUS THROMBOSIS
See **Table 7-1**.

Table 7-1. Medical Conditions or Disorders Associated With Superior Sagittal Sinus Thrombosis in Infants and Children
— Acute tonsillitis with abscess and central nervous system complications
— Anticoagulant drug therapy complications
— Behçet disease in adolescents with increased intracranial pressure
— Birth asphyxia and cerebral infarction in neonates with seizures
— Dehydration with severe hypernatremia
— Epidural abscess with central nervous system extension
— Frontal bone osteomyelitis and central nervous system extension
— Homocystinuria with antithrombin III and factor VII deficiencies
— Leukemia with dural sinus occlusion
— Nephrotic syndrome *(continued)*

Table 7-1. *(continued)*

— Oral contraceptive pills

— Pregnancy and early postpartum stages in the adolescent mother (both can lead to hypercoagulability)

— Protein C or S deficiency

— Sinusitis with paranasal extension of abscess

— Systemic malignancy with central nervous system metastasis

— Thrombotic events related to indwelling catheters

— Traumatic brain injury

ACCIDENTAL AND WITNESSED INJURIES CAUSING INTRACRANIAL HEMORRHAGE

— *Intraventricular hemorrhage in neonates.* Differentiate by history and radiology.

— *Traumatic aneurysm of the middle meningeal artery.* Differentiate by history and radiology.

— *Caida de mollera (fallen fontanel).* Folk remedy. Differentiate by history and physical examination.

— *Breakdancing.* Seen in adolescents. Differentiate by history and physical examination.

— *Headbanging to music.* Seen in adolescents. Differentiate by history.

— *Roller coaster rides.* Differentiate by history.

— *Ute surfing.* Australian pastime involving riding on the load tray of a moving sport utitlty vehicle, often after consuming alcohol. Seen in adolescents. Differentiate by history.

— *Tangential missile wound to the head.* Differentiate by history and physical examination.

— *Boxing.* Seen in adolescents and adults. Differentiate by history.

— *Valsalva maneuver.* With heavy weight lifting, is reported only in adults. Differentiate by history.

GENETIC AND METABOLIC DISORDERS
— Assessment is guided by 3 principles:

1. Broad screening for every disorder in every case is not warranted. Use history, physical examination, imaging, and appropriate screening tests to guide diagnosis. Monitor clinical course.

2. The incidence rates of most of these diseases in childhood are much lower than for common pediatric illnesses and child abuse. Diagnosis must include coordinated evaluations with pediatric subspecialists.

3. Diagnosis of a genetic or metabolic disorder can coexist with child abuse.

— *Sickle cell anemia.* Differentiate by history and laboratory tests.

— *Osteogenesis imperfecta.*[23,24] Vascular fragility, skull deformity, skull fracture, or associated conditions predispose to SDH with or without trauma. Differentiate by history, physical examination, radiology, and laboratory tests.

— *Ehlers-Danlos syndrome.* Differentiate by history, physical examination, and laboratory tests.

— *Marfan syndrome.*[25] Collagen defect and vascular fragility may cause aneurysm and bleeding. Differentiate by history and physical examination.

— *Menkes kinky hair syndrome.* Caused by a defective gene that regulates the metabolism of copper. Brain atrophy can cause SDH. Differentiate by history, physical examination, radiology, and laboratory tests.

— *Autosomal dominant polycystic kidney disease.* Differentiate by history and radiology.

— *Incontinentia pigmenti.*[26] A rare disease involving cerebral infarct, edema, and hemorrhagic white matter encephalopathy. Differentiate by history, physical examination, radiology, and laboratory tests.

— *Alagille syndrome.*[27,28] Thinness of the skull may predispose to intracranial epidural hemorrhage or bleeding may result from hypercholesterolemia or defective hemostatic function. Differentiate by history, physical examination, radiology, and laboratory tests.

— *Glutaricaciduria type I.* See **Figure 7-2**. Differentiate by history, physical examination, radiology, and laboratory tests.

— *Galactosemia.* Differentiate by history and laboratory tests.

— *Homocystinuria.*[29,30] Possibly associated with antithrombin III or factor VI deficiency and subsequent superior sagittal sinus thrombosis

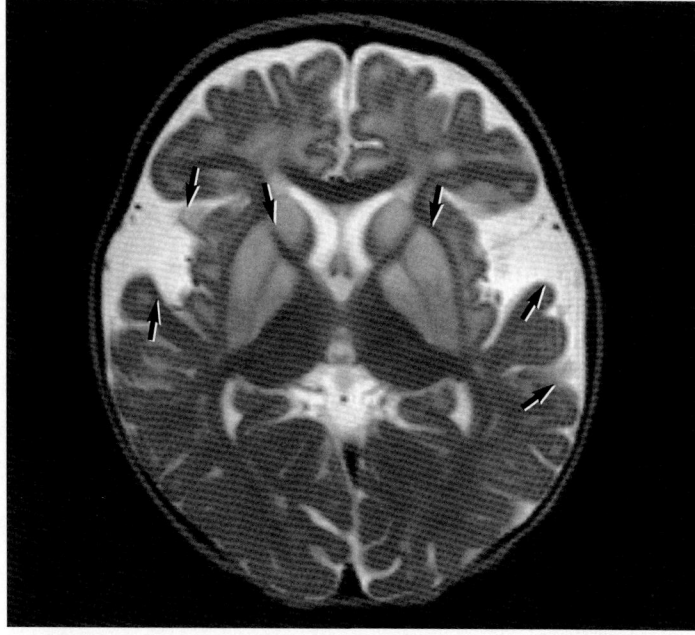

Figure 7-2. *Magnetic resonance imaging (MRI) scan of 16-month-old girl showing abnormal increased T2 signals in the bilateral basal ganglia and increased periventricular T2 white-matter signals (arrows) with cortical volume loss. These findings are consistent with glutaricaciduria type I (glutaryl-CoA dehydrogenase deficiency).*

(SSST). Differentiate by history, physical examination, radiology, and laboratory tests.

— *Cerebral ceroidosis in albinos*. Differentiate by history, physical examination, radiology, and laboratory tests.

— *Hyperostosis frontalis interna*.[31] A rare condition causing frontal bossing in adults. Differentiate by history, physical examination, and radiology.

HEMATOLOGICAL DISEASES AND DISORDERS OF COAGULATION AND CLOTTING

— *Hemorrhagic disease of the newborn*.[32] Caused by vitamin K deficiency at birth and involves early and late manifestations with SDH. Differentiate by history, radiology, and laboratory tests.

— *Hemophilia A (factor VIII deficiency) and B (factor IX deficiency)*. See **Figure 7-3**. Differentiate by history and physical examination.

— *Factor V deficiency (parahemophilia)*. Differentiate by history, physical examination, and laboratory tests.

— *Factor XII deficiency*. Differentiate by history, physical examination, and laboratory tests.

— *von Willebrand disease*. SDH reported in older children, not infants. Differentiate by history, physical examination, and laboratory tests.

— *Congenital dysfibrinogenemia*.[33] A rare inherited fibrinogen disorder. Differentiate by history, physical examination, and laboratory tests.

— *Idiopathic thrombocytopenia purpura*.[34] May be idiopathic or drug-induced. Differentiate by history and laboratory tests.

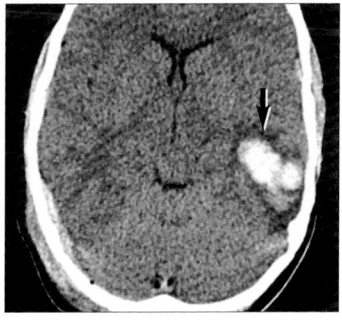

Figure 7-3. *Noncontrast CT scan of 10-year-old boy with hemophilia A showing a large acute left temporal parenchymal hematoma (arrow), a small right occipital subdural-versus-epidural hematoma, and early cerebral edema.*

— *Disseminated intravascular coagulation.*[35] Can be associated with cancer, infection, or trauma. Differentiate by history, physical examination, and laboratory tests.

— *Cirrhosis-of-liver-induced coagulopathy.*[36] Impairs clotting factor production. Differentiate by history, physical examination, and laboratory tests.

— *Acquired inhibitors of plasma clotting factors.* Differentiate by history and laboratory tests.

— *Anticoagulant therapies.* Differentiate by history, physical examination, and laboratory tests.

— *Lupus anticoagulant.* Differentiate by history and laboratory tests.

— *Antiphospholipid antibody syndrome.* Differentiate by history and laboratory tests.

INFECTIOUS DISEASES

— Hemophilus influenzae *and* Streptococcus pneumoniae *meningitis.*[37] Can cause subdural effusions resembling chronic SDHs. Differentiate by history, physical examination, radiology, and laboratory tests.

— *Other bacterial meningitis pathogens.*[38] Subdural effusions are less common with *Neisseria meningitides*, group B *Streptococcus, Escherichia coli,* and *Listeria.* Differentiate by history, physical examination, radiology, and laboratory tests.

— *Herpes encephalitis.*[39,40] Devastating central nervous system (CNS) hemorrhage is possible (**Figures 7-4-a** and **b**). Differentiate by history, physical examination, and laboratory tests.

— *Chronic otitis media*[41,42] *and sinusitis.*[43] Produce subdural effusions and empyema resembling chronic SDHs. Differentiate by history, physical examination, and laboratory tests.

— *Acute tonsillitis.*[44] Involves parapharyngeal abscess with CNS complication and sinus thrombosis. Differentiate by history, physical examination, radiology, and laboratory tests.

— *Malaria.* Differentiate by history and laboratory tests.

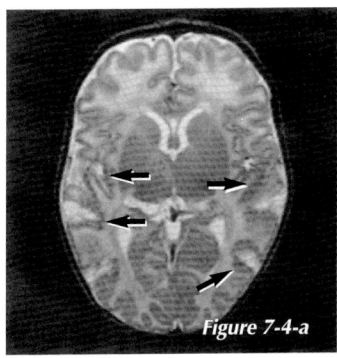 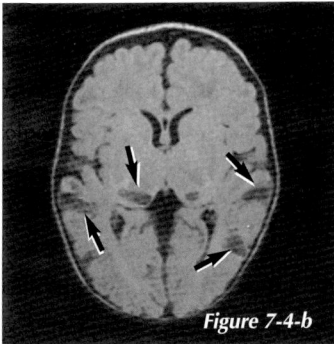

Figure 7-4-a. *Gadolinium-contrast MRI head scan of 1-week-old febrile infant. Menin-geal enhancement in the right temporal and bilateral posterior parietal and occipital regions (arrows) is consistent with meningitis.*

Figure 7-4-b. *Subsequent gadolinium-contrast MRI head scan shows multifocal bilateral parietal, temporal, and thalamic infarctions that developed into encephalomalacia within 1 month (arrows).*

— *Congenital toxoplasmosis.* Differentiate by history, physical examination, radiology, and laboratory tests.

— *Ruptured mycotic aneurysm from bacterial endocarditis.*[45] Occurs in adult women, with possible complications in children. Differentiate by history, radiology, and laboratory tests.

— *Encephalopathy of infancy and childhood.*[46] Can be caused by infection; postinfection hypoxic conditions; or toxic, metabolic, or idiopathic factors. Differentiate by history, physical examination, radiology, and laboratory tests.

AUTOIMMUNE AND VASCULITIC CONDITIONS

— *Systemic lupus erythematosus.* Differentiate by history, physical examination, and laboratory tests.

— *Kawasaki disease.*[47,48] Subdural effusions (not hemorrhages) occur secondary to leptomeningeal vasculitis. Differentiate by history, physical examination, and laboratory tests.

— *Moyamoya disease.*[49] A rare vascular disease. Differentiate by radiology.

— *Wegener granulomatosis.* Differentiate by history, radiology, and laboratory tests.

— *Behçet disease.*[50] Increased ICP results from SSST and occurs in adolescent males. Differentiate by history, physical examination, radiology, and laboratory tests.

ONCOLOGICAL DISEASES

— *Leukemia.* Differentiate by history, physical examination, and laboratory tests.

— *Solid CNS tumors.* Differentiate by history, physical examination, radiology, and laboratory tests.

— *Lymphoma in dura mater.* Differentiate by laboratory tests.

— *Subdural sarcoma.* Differentiate by radiology.

— *Meningioma.* Differentiate by history, physical examination, radiology, and laboratory tests.

— *Choroid plexus carcinoma and papilloma.*[51] Are rare intraventricular tumors. Differentiate by history, physical examination, radiology, and laboratory tests.

— *Systemic nonprimary malignancy.* Differentiate by history, radiology, and laboratory tests.

— *Meningeal metastases.* Differentiate by history, physical examination, radiology, and laboratory tests.

— *Giant xanthogranulomas.*[52] Are rare in children. Differentiate by history, radiology, and laboratory tests.

— *Cancer therapy.*[53] Can result in hematologic and coagulation defects, opportunistic infections associated with bleeding, and bleeding caused by radiation treatments. Differentiate by history, physical examination, radiology, and laboratory tests.

— *Tamoxifen.* Differentiate by history and physical examination.

TOXINS, POISONS, AND NUTRITIONAL DEFICIENCIES

— *Lead poisoning.* Differentiate by history, radiology, and laboratory tests.

— *Ginkgo biloba ingestions.* Differentiate by history, physical examination, and laboratory tests.

— *Cocaine use.* Differentiate by history and laboratory tests.

— *Brodifacoum (rat poison) ingestion.* Differentiate by history, physical examination, and laboratory tests.

— *Vitamin K deficiency, hemorrhagic disease of the newborn, rickets, liver disease, or liver failure in children.* Differentiate by history, radiology, and laboratory tests (**Figure 7-5-a** and **b**).

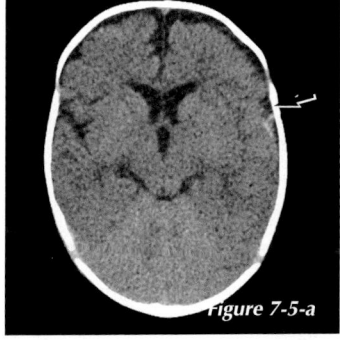

Figure 7-5-a. *CT scan of child with rickets demonstrating small, localized subarachnoid hemorrhage (arrow).*

Figure 7-5-b. *CT scan of same child demonstrating an orbital hematoma (arrow).*

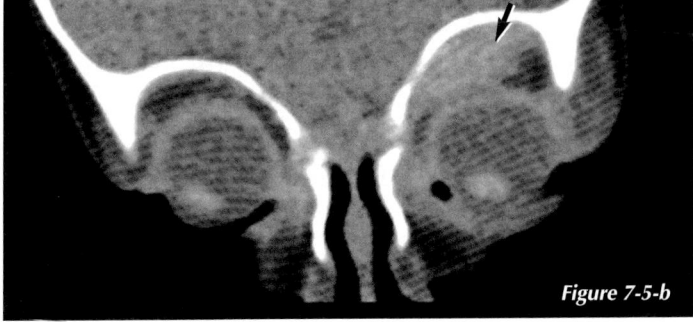

Figure 7-5-b

— *Scurvy*. Differentiate by history, physical examination, radiology, and laboratory tests.

MEDICAL AND SURGICAL COMPLICATIONS

— *Anticoagulant therapies*. Differentiate by history, physical examination, and laboratory tests.

— *Spinal tap*. Differentiate by history.

— *Spinal anesthesia*. Differentiate by history.

— *Epidural anesthesia*. Differentiate by history.

— *Lumbar myelography*. Differentiate by history.

— *Subdural taps*. Differentiate by history and physical examination.

— *Intrathecal injection*. Differentiate by history, physical examination, and radiology.

— *Ventriculoperitoneal or ventriculoarterial shunts*. Differentiate by history, physical examination, and radiology.

— *Epilepsy surgery*. Differentiate by history, physical examination, and radiology.

— *Subdural fat effusion after parenteral nutrition*. Differentiate by history and physical examination.

— *Oral surgery complication*. Differentiate by history, physical examination, and radiology.

— *Anticoagulant therapy in prosthetic valve patients*.[54] Reported only in adults. Differentiate by history, physical examination, and laboratory tests.

— *Hemodialysis*. Differentiate by history and physical examination.

— *Liver transplant*. Differentiate by history, physical examination, radiology, and laboratory tests.

— *Open heart surgery*.[55] Rarely reported and possibly related to anticoagulation or cerebral blood flow changes with the bypass. Differentiate by history and physical examination.

— *Low-dose adrenal corticotrophin hormone therapy for infantile spasms*. Differentiate by history and physical examination.

REFERENCES

1. Zalneraitis EL, Young RS, Krishnamoorthy KS. Intracranial hemorrhage in utero as a complication of isoimmune thrombocytopenia. *J Pediatr.* 1979;95:611-614.

2. Gunn TR, Mok PM, Becroft DM. Sudural hemorrhage in utero. *Pediatrics.* 1985;76:605-610.

3. Hankins GD, Leicht T, Van Hook J, Uckan EM. The role of forceps rotation in maternal and neonatal injury. *Am J Obstet Gynecol.* 1999;180(pt1):231-234.

4. Hanigan WC, Morgan AM, Stahlberg LK, Hiller JL. Tentorial hemorrhage associated with vacuum extraction. *Pediatrics.* 1990;85:534-539.

5. Abroms IF, McLennan JE, Mandell F. Acute neonatal subdural hematoma following breech delivery. *Am J Dis Child.* 1977;131:192-194.

6. Govaert P, Vanhaesebrouck P, de Praeter C. Traumatic neonatal intracranial bleeding and stroke. *Arch Dis Child.* 1992;67:840-845.

7. Bills DC, Rosenfeld JV, Phelan EM, Klug GL. Intracranial arteriovenous malformations in childhood: presentation, management, and outcome. *J Clin Neurosci.* 1996;3:220-228.

8. Allison JW, Davis PC, Sato Y, et al. Intracranial aneurysms in infants and children. *Pediatr Radiol.* 1998;28:223-229.

9. Kanaan I, Lasjaunias P, Coates R. The spectrum on intracranial aneurysm in pediatrics. *Minim Invasive Neurosurg.* 1995;38:1-9.

10. O'Leary PM, Sweeny PJ. Ruptured intracerebral aneurysms in a subdural hematoma. *Ann Emerg Med.* 1986;15:944-946.

11. Belzic I, Yaseen H, Voirin J, Bonte JB, Laloum D. Cerebral arteriovenous malformations in a probable familial form of Rendu-Osler disease [in French]. *Ann Pediatr (Paris).* 1992;39:301-304.

12. Roy C, Noseda G, Arzimanoglou A, et al. Rendu Osler disease revealed by ruptured cerebral arterial aneurysm in an infant [in French]. *Arch Fr Pediatr.* 1990;47:741-742.

13. Romero FJ, Rovira M Jr, Ibarra B, Piqueras J, Rovira M. Arachnoid cysts with intracystic and subdural haematoma. *Eur J Radiol.* 1989; 9:119-120.

14. Robinson MJ, Cameron MD, Smith MF, Ayers AB. Fetal subdural haemorrhages presenting as hydrocephalus. *Br Med J.* 1980;281:35.

15. Jiminez DF, Barone CM. Encephaloceles, meningoceles, and dermal sinusus. In: Alright L, Pollack I, Adelson D, eds. *Principles and Practices of Pediatric Neurosurgery.* New York, NY: Thieme Medical Publishers; 1999:189-208.

16. Ceccherini AF, Jaspan T. Cerebral herniation through a subdural membrane defect following non-accidental injury. *Clin Radiol.* 1999;54:550-552.

17. David S, Salluzzo RF, Bartfield JM, Dickinson ET. Spontaneous cervicothoracic epidural hematoma following prolonged Valsalva secondary to trumpet playing. *Am J Emerg Med.* 1997;15:73-75.

18. Newton RW. Intracranial hemorrhage and non-accidental injury. *Arch Dis Child.* 1989;64:188-190.

19. deVeber G, Andrew M, Adams C, et al. Cerebral sinovenous thrombosis in children. *N Engl J Med.* 2001;345:417-423.

20. de Villiers R, Kuyler J. Superior sagittal sinus thrombosis. *S Afr Med J.* 2000;90:481.

21. Divekar AA, Ali US, Ronghe MD, Singh AR, Dalvi RB. Superior sagittal sinus thrombosis in a child with nephrotic syndrome. *Pediatr Nephrol.* 1996;10:206-207.

22. Imai WK, Everhart FR Jr, Sanders JM Jr. Cerebral venous sinus thrombosis: report of a case and review of the literature [review]. *Pediatrics.* 1982;70:965-970.

23. Cole WG, Lam TP. Arachnoid cyst and chronic subdural haematoma in a child with osteogenesis imperfecta type III resulting from the substitution of glycine 1006 by alanine in the pro alpha 2(I) chain of type I procollagen. *J Med Genet.* 1996;33:193-196.

24. Sayre MR, Roberge RJ, Evans TC. Nontraumatic subdural hematoma in a patient with osteogenesis imperfecta and renal failure. *Am J Emerg Med*. 1987;5:298-301.

25. Buchanan R, Wyatt GP. Marfan's syndrome presenting as an intrapartum death. *Arch Dis Child*. 1985;60:1074-1076.

26. Ciarallo L, Paller AS. Two cases of incontinentia pigmenti simulating child abuse. *Pediatrics*. 1997;100:e6.

27. Woolfenden AR, Albers GW, Steinberg GK, Hahn JS, Johnston DC, Farrell K. Moyamoya syndrome in children with Alagille syndrome: additional evidence of a vasculopathy. *Pediatrics*. 1999;101:505-508.

28. Lykavieris P, Crosnier C, Trichet C, Meunier-Rotival M, Hadchouel M. Bleeding tendency in children with Alagille syndrome. *Pediatrics*. 2003;111:167-170.

29. Cochran FB, Sweetman L, Schmidt K, Barsh G, Kraus J, Packman S. Pyridoxine-unresponsive homocystinuria with an unusual clinical course. *Am J Med Genet*. 1990;35:519-522.

30. Kang HS, Kim DG, Yoon BW. Superior sagittal sinus thrombosis with homocystinuria and deficiency of antithrombin III and factor VII: case report. *Acta Neurochir (Wien)*. 1998;140:196-198.

31. Ishiguro M, Nakagawa T, Yamamura N, Kurokawa Y. Japanese cases of hyperostosis frontalis interna [in Japanese]. *No To Shinkei*. 1997;49:899-904.

32. Rutty GN, Smith CM, Malia RG. Late-form hemorrhagic disease of the newborn: a fatal case report with illustration of investigations that may assist in avoiding the mistaken diagnosis of child abuse. *Am J Forensic Med Pathol*. 1999;20:48-51.

33. al-Fawaz IM, Gader AM. Severe congenital dysfibrinogenemia (fibrinogen-Riyadh): a family study. *Acta Haematol*. 1992;33:194-197.

34. Kolluri VR, Reddy DR, Reddy PK, Naidu MR, Kumari CS. Subdural hematoma secondary to immune thrombocytopenic purpura: a case report. *Neurosurgery*. 1986;10:635-636.

35. Furui T, Ichihara K, Ikeda A, et al. Subdural hematoma associated with disseminated intravascular coagulation in patients with advanced cancer. *J Neurosurg.* 1983;58:398-401.

36. Furui T, Yamada A, Iwata K. Subdural hematoma as a complication of hemostatic deficiency secondary to liver cirrhosis—report of two cases. *Neurol Med Child (Tokyo).* 1989;29:588-591.

37. Ogilvy CS, Chapman PH, McGrail K. Subdural empyema complicating bacterial meningitis in a child: enhancement of membranes with gadolinium on magnetic resonance imaging in a patient without enhancement on computed tomography. *Surg Neurol.* 1992; 37:137-141.

38. Syrogiannopoulos GA, Nelson JD, McCracken GH Jr. Subdural collections of fluid in acute bacterial meningitis: a review of 136 cases. *Pediatr Infect Dis.* 1986;5:343-352.

39. Fenton LZ, Sirotnak AP, Handler MH. Parietal pseudofracture and spontaneous intracranial hemorrhage suggesting nonaccidental trauma: report of 2 cases. *Pediatr Neurosurg.* 2000;33:318-322.

40. Henter JI, Nennesmo I. Neuropathologic findings and neurologic symptoms in twenty-three children with hemophagocytic lymphohistiocytosis. *Pediatrics.* 1997;130:358-365.

41. Gower D, McGuirt WF. Intracranial complications of acute and chronic infectious ear disease: a problem still with us. *Laryngoscope.* 1983;93:1028-1033.

42. Gower D, McGuirt WF, Kelly DL Jr. Intracranial complications of ear disease in a pediatric population with special emphasis on subdural effusion and empyema. *South Med J.* 1985;78:429-434.

43. Gallagher RM, Gross CW, Phillips CD. Suppurative intracranial complications of sinusitis. *Laryngoscope.* 1998;108(pt 1):1635-1642.

44. Morgan N, Brookes GB. Central nervous system complications of acute tonsillitis. *J Laryngol Otol.* 1997;111:274-276.

45. Bandoh K, Sugimura J, Hosaka Y, Takagi S. Ruptured intracranial

mycotic aneurysm associated with acute subdural hematoma—case report. *Neurol Med Chir (Tokyo)*. 1987;27:56-59.

46. Haslam RA. Encephalopathies. In: Behrman RE, Kliegman RM, Jenson HB, eds. *Nelson Textbook of Pediatrics*. 16th ed. Philadelphia, Pa: WB Saunders; 2000.

47. Akoi N. Subdural effusion in the acute stage of Kawsaki disease. *Surg Neurol*. 1988;29:216-217.

48. Fujiwara S, Yamano T, Hattori M, Fujiseki Y, Shimada M. Asymptomatic cerebral infarction in Kawasaki disease. *Pediatr Neurol*. 1992;8:235-236.

49. Takeuchi S, Ichikawa A, Koike T, Tanaka R, Arai H. Acute subdural hematoma in young patient with moyamoya disease—case report. *Neurol Med Child (Tokyo)*. 1992;32:80-83.

50. Stern JM, Kesler SM. Raised intracranial pressure in a 16-year-old boy. Report of a case of Behçet's disease. *S Afr Med J*. 1989;75:243-244.

51. Pencalet P, Sainte-Rose C, Lellouch-Tubiana A, et al. Papillomas and carcinomas of the choroid plexus in children. *J Neurosurg*. 1998;88:521-528.

52. Gaskill SJ, Saldivar V, Rutman J, Marlin AE. Giant bilateral xathogranulomas in a child: case report. *Neurosurgery*. 1992;31:114-117.

53. Graus F, Rogers LR, Posner JB. Cerebrovascular complications in patients with cancer. *Medicine (Baltimore)*. 1985;64:16-35.

54. Nakagawa T, Kubota T, Handa Y, Kawano H, Sato K. Intracranial hemorrhage due to long-term anticoagulant therapy in prosthetic heart valves—four case reports. *Neurol Med Chir (Tokyo)*. 1995;35:156-159.

55. Yokote H, Itakura T, Funahashi K, Kamei I, Hayashi S, Komai N. Chronic subdural hematoma after open heart surgery. *Surg Neurol*. 1985;24:520-524.

8

NURSING CARE

Leslie K. Pfeil, RN, BSN, CCRN(P)

EMERGENCY MANAGEMENT

Recognize the symptoms of mild, moderate, and severe abusive head trauma (AHT) (see Chapter 1, Recognizing Intentional and Unintentional Head Injuries).

STABILIZE AIRWAY, BREATHING, AND CARDIOVASCULAR STATUS

— Cervical spine precautions:

1. If the patient is apneic, has insufficient respiratory effort, and respiratory therapy is not available, perform jaw-thrust maneuvers and begin bag-valve-mask (BVM) ventilations with 100% oxygen while other personnel institute full cervical spine precautions. This includes use of a cervical collar, head blocks, and a rigid board with appropriately fitted straps (**Table 8-1** and **Appendix 8-1**).

2. Employ 2 to 4 people to adequately protect the cervical spine while instituting precautions.

Table 8-1. Symptoms of Mild to Moderate Abusive Head Trauma	
— Irritability	— Increased or decreased muscle tone
— Vomiting	— Increasing head size
— Feeding difficulties	— Failure to thrive
— Lethargy	— Facial brusing
— Drowsiness	— Excessive crying

3. Assume that all patients with suspected AHT have a cervical spine injury until proved otherwise.

4. Maintain strict cervical spine precautions throughout all procedures, including intubation.

— Ventilations and pulse:

1. Start BVM ventilations, then observe the patient's chest rise to determine whether ventilations are adequate.

2. Palpate for a pulse in a central location.

   A. Infants and children: brachial or femoral

   B. Neonates: umbilicus

3. If the patient does not have a pulse, immediately initiate cardiopulmonary resuscitation following standardized Pediatric Advanced Life Support algorithms.

4. Have additional nursing personnel place the patient on continous monitoring equipment (electrocardiogram [ECG], respiratory machines, and pulse oximetry).

OTHER MEASURES
— Place an intravenous (IV) line for the purposes of blood sampling and the administration of emergency and anticonvulsant medications and fluid resuscitation.

1. Anticonvulsant medications are needed if seizures are suspected. Seizures occur in 40% to 70% of patients with inflicted head injuries.

2. Establish intraosseous (IO) infusion quickly if the first few IV attempts are unsuccessful or if IV access is unlikely.[1]

   A. Although any resuscitation fluid, medication, or blood product can be given through an IO needle, IO infusion requires more pressure, which is obtained using an infusion pump, manual blood pressure (BP) cuff, pressure bag, or by pushing the fluid with a syringe.

    B. Watch IO entrance site and surrounding tissue carefully and monitor frequently for infiltration.

— Perform a secondary survey to identify added injuries.

— Perform a computed tomography scan to determine if immediate surgery is needed.

— Transfer the child to the pediatric intensive care unit (PICU) or pediatric trauma center.

— File a report of suspected abuse with the appropriate authorities.

INTENSIVE CARE MANAGEMENT

— The goal of PICU care is to prevent secondary brain injury while supporting vital functions.

— Patients initially diagnosed with AHT are likely to worsen as time passes because cerebral edema generally progresses for 48 to 72 hours after the initial event.

INITIAL MEASURES

— Include endotracheal tube (ETT) placement, evaluation of central versus peripheral pulses, capillary refill, and IV line patency in rapid assessment of airway, breathing, and circulation.

— Complete the baseline neurological examination while the patient is connected to continuous ECG and pulse oximetry monitoring devices.

— Take BP frequently.

— Keep suction equipment and BVM with an appropriately sized mask and continuous flow of 100% oxygen readily available.

— Ensure adequate and secure IV access.

— Review laboratory values obtained by the emergency department or referring institution.

— Send blood or other body fluids for testing as indicated.

— Place a nasogastric tube unless confirmed or suspected basilar skull fractures are present. With these fractures, place an orogastric tube.

— Place a Foley catheter to maintain strict intake and output records.

— Patients need to have 1 assigned nurse, with other nurses as backup support until initial procedures are completed and stable condition is achieved.

— Record vital signs and neurological examination results hourly.

— If neuroradiological imaging was not previously obtained, do so as soon as the patient's condition permits to evaluate the need for surgery.

RESPIRATORY INTERVENTIONS

— Airway and cervical spine management remain priorities upon admission to the PICU.

— Respiratory assessment: Document respiratory rate, breathing sounds, oxygen saturation, possible increased work of breathing (presence of nasal flaring, retractions, grunting, and extraneous airway noise).

— If the patient needs extensive radiological assessment, intubate to maintain control of the airway and to avoid emergency intubation during procedures.

— If the patient is intubated, confirm proper endotracheal position by observing equal chest rise, auscultating for equal breath sounds, detecting end tidal carbon dioxide level, and obtaining a chest radiograph.

— Additional assessments: Note the location and landmarks of the ETT, the security of the ETT, ventilatory settings, and airway pressure readings.

— Maintain partial pressure of carbon dioxide in arterial blood ($PaCO_2$) between 35 and 38 mm Hg and oxygen saturation greater than or equal to 92%.

— Avoid hyperventilation in children with traumatic brain injury because it produces brain ischemia.[2]

— Avoid high peak pressures and positive end expiratory pressures because they can decrease cerebral venous return.[3]

CARDIOVASCULAR INTERVENTIONS

— Cardiovascular assessment: Document the patient's heart rate, BP, quality of central versus peripheral pulses, central and peripheral capillary refill, skin color, skin temperature, and hourly urine output.

— The patient may require continuous dopamine infusion and/or epinephrine infusion to maintain normal BP and adequate perfusion.

— Patients often develop disseminated intravascular coagulopathy (DIC), which requires multiple transfusions of various types of blood products.[4]

NEUROLOGICAL INTERVENTIONS

— Neurological evaluation:

1. Assess level of consciousness using a consistent rating scale such as the modified Glasgow Coma Scale (**Table 8-2**).

Table 8-2. Modified Glasgow Coma Scale for Infants and Children

	CHILD	INFANT	SCORE
Eye opening	Spontaneous	Spontaneous	4
	To verbal stimuli	To verbal stimuli	3
	To pain only	To pain only	2
	No response	No response	1
Verbal response	Oriented, appropriate	Coos and babbles	5
	Confused	Irritable cries	4
	Inappropriate words	Cries to pain	3
	Incomprehensible words or nonspecific sounds	Moans to pain	2
	No response	No response	1

(continued)

Table 8-2. *(continued)*

	CHILD	INFANT	SCORE
Motor response	Obeys commands	Moves spontaneously and purposefully	6
	Localizes painful stimuli	Withdraws to touch	5
	Withdraws in response to pain	Withdraws in response to pain	4
	Flexion in response to pain	Decorticate posturing (abnormal flexion) in response to pain	3
	Extension in response to pain	Decerebrate posturing (abnormal extension) in response to pain	2
	No response	No response	1

Adapted from Teasdale,[5] with permission from Elsevier.

2. Measure the patient's eye opening, motor, and verbal responses.

— Check that pupils are equal in size and respond equally to light.

— Observe for consensual pupil constriction.

— Be familiar with medications that affect pupil size and the duration of these medications.

1. Opiates constrict pupils and may be given when the child is intubated.

2. Atropine and high doses of dopamine dilate pupils.

— Notify physician:

1. If pupils remain dilated and nonreactive to light after the medication's effectiveness is over.

2. If pupils are unequal in size or unresponsive to light (1 or both).

— Evaluate movement and sensation in extremities.

1. Assess spontaneous and purposeful movement in response to pain rather than reflexive responses.

2. Purposeful movement can be assessed by applying a central pain stimulus to the head, neck, or chest.

3. Notify the physician of diminished response, decorticate or decerebrate posture, or flaccid extremities if these differ from the previous findings.

— Obtain daily head circumference measurements in infants.

— If the anterior fontanel is still open, assess for fullness, bulging, and pulsations.[6]

Pressure Monitoring
— Intracranial pressure (ICP)

1. ICP is a critical vital sign to detect and manage secondary brain injury.

2. Measure ICP via catheter or pressure-sensitive fiber device inserted into a burr hole created in the skull and positioned at various depths in the meninges-brain-ventricular anatomy, then transduce the fluid column pressure or electrical signal to the bedside monitor.

3. The pressure within this system is compared to atmospheric pressure and is displayed on a continuous readout (**Table 8-3**).

Table 8-3. Signs and Symptoms of Increased Intracranial Pressure in Children

CHANGE IN LEVEL OF CONSCIOUSNESS

Irritability then lethargy

Confusion, disorientation

Decreased responsiveness (decreased eye contact; decreased response to parent and pain)

Reduced ability to follow commands (eg, to hold up 2 fingers, wiggle toes, stick out tongue)   *(continued)*

Table 8-3. *(continued)*

PUPIL DIALATION WITH DECREASED RESPONSE TO LIGHT

REDUCED SPONTANEOUS MOVEMENT OR DETERIORATION IN REFLEXIVE POSTURING

> Purposeful movement deterioration
>
> Decorticate posture, then . . .
>
> Decerebrate posture, then . . .
>
> Flaccid response to pain

CUSHING'S TRIAD (HYPERTENSION, BRADYCARDIA, APNEA): MAY OCCUR ONLY AS LATE SIGN

Adapted from Hazinski,[7] with permission from Elsevier.

---

4. Normal ICP range is 4 to 15 mm Hg.[3]

5. ***Hypertension*** is an ICP greater than 20 mm Hg that lasts more than 5 minutes. Report this level to the physician so interventions can be taken to lower ICP.

— Cerebral perfusion pressure (CPP) and mean arterial pressure (MAP)

1. CPP is calculated by subtracting the ICP from the MAP.

2. Determine the MAP from arterial line rather than manual or automatic BP cuff.

3. Maintain CPP of at least 50 mm Hg with traumatic brain injury, except in infants and toddlers. Regardless of age, CPP greater than 40 mm Hg is associated with increased mortality.

4. CPP decreases with rises in ICP, fall in BP, or both simultaneously.

5. To treat low CPP, increase BP, decrease ICP, or both.

6. CPP is not an absolute indicator of cerebral perfusion because it is determined by cerebral blood flow, not overall BP.

7. Normal CPP does not necessarily indicate normal cerebral blood flow.

— Cushing's triad

1. Configuration of symptoms signifying an increased ICP.

2. Consists of bradycardia, increased systolic BP with widening pulse pressure (hypertension), and apnea.

3. Appearance typically indicates that significantly elevated ICP is already present and cerebral herniation is impending.

4. Is often preceded by tachycardia and fluctuating BP.

5. If the patient's heart rate unexpectedly rises above baseline and BP becomes labile, perform rapid neurological assessment and notify the physician.

— Effect of environment and medical interventions:

1. ICP rises with turning, suctioning, and venipuncture.

2. Space these activities out to prevent cumulative effect.

3. Apply topical anesthetics or use parenteral systemic analgesics or sedatives to blunt response.

4. Protect the patient from adverse stimuli, including family visits if these increase ICP.

   A. Gently explain the situation to the family.

   B. Offer a place to sit and observe in the patient's room without interacting directly.

5. Encourage environmental stimulation that improves ICP, such as soft music or family visits.

— Seizure activity:

1. Increases ICP and must be recognized and treated quickly.

2. Signs include pupil dilation, fluctuating vital signs, sucking motions, lip smacking, rhythmic twitching in any extremity, and sudden neurological deterioration.[6] The signs can be subtle in infants.

3.   Subclinical seizures may only be evident on electroencephalogram.

4.   Notify the physician when seizure activity occurs.

5.   Observe and record the type of seizure, where the seizures begin, where they extend, how long they last, and whether they affect vital signs.

6.   After anticonvulsant medications are given, monitor and document response.

7.   It is a misconception that infants tolerate increased ICP better than older children because their fontanel is open or sutures can split to allow room for swelling.

   A.   The dura mater encasing the brain is inelastic with no allowance for rapid expansion.

   B.   Infants have shorter spinal cords and therefore less room to displace blood and cerebrospinal fluid.

   C.   ICP increases with a 5 mm fluid increase in infants; adolescents suffer similar ICP increase only with 3 times this much fluid.

Treatment for Increased ICP
— Elevated levels may occur in the first hours after PICU admission even if not present on admission.

— The goal is to restore and optimize CPP.

— Elevate the head of the bed 30 degrees.

— Fix the child's head and neck in straight alignment. This position is highly recommended for children with increased ICP caused by AHT.

— Osmotic agents and diuretics may alter volume status.

1.   Includes mannitol (osmotic agent) and hypertonic 3% sodium chloride.

2.   Schedule frequent tests of serum sodium and osmolality.

3.   Follow the physician's parameters for discontinuation.[2]

4.   Monitor electrolytes for developing syndrome of inappropriate antidiuretic hormone or diabetes insipidus (DI). Both can induce

rapid changes in serum sodium level or osmolality, causing free water to shift and contribute to cerebral edema.

Pharmacological Paralysis

— Creates a challenge for the nurse to adequately assess level of sedation and level of muscular block to ensure the patient is properly sedated while chemically paralyzed.

— Risks of neuromuscular blockade (NMB) include hypoxia secondary to inadvertent displacement of ETT, masking seizures, increased rate of nosocomial pneumonia, cardiovascular effects, immobilization stress.[8]

— If patients are not sufficiently sedated (awake paralysis), they may experience anxiety and pain, which increase heart rate, BP, and metabolic demands.

— Can develop posttraumatic stress after discharge.

— Heart rate, BP, level of diaphoresis, and tearing are not reliable (may be manifestations of underlying disease processes).[9]

— Monitoring the level of NMB:

1. The Food and Drug Administration recommends a peripheral nerve stimulator (PNS), which delivers a small electrical stimulus (usually applied to wrist) to a nerve that stimulates a muscle contraction.

2. Only the train-of-four setting on the PNS is used in the critical care setting; assess regularly.[10]

3. Treat anxiety and pain aggressively to avoid increasing ICP.

4. Control fever with antipyretics because it increases cerebral blood flow and cerebral metabolic rate.

5. Begin nutritional support within 72 hours; use full replacement in 7 days.[11]

6. Consult rehabilitation service personnel early in the treatment process to begin the process of assisting with musculoskeletal deficits.

DOCUMENTATION

— Health care professionals are required by law to report suspected child abuse to appropriate authorities in accordance with each state's provisions.

— Types of documentation: written forms, diagrams, photographs

— Must be detailed, accurate, and objective.[12]

— It is best to have the most experienced health care professionals record injuries to ensure documentation is accurate and valuable to investigators and the judicial system.

— Hospital-based suspected child abuse and neglect (SCAN) teams can provide assistance.

1. The team includes physicians specially trained in child abuse evaluation, nurse practitioners, nurses, social workers, and chaplains.

2. The team's goal is to provide a comprehensive assessment and recommendations for treatment of suspected child abuse.

3. Contact the SCAN team early in the process of properly documenting and evaluating a case and obtain consultations as needed.

4. In the absence of such a team, medical teams or law enforcement agencies document the findings.

— Use accurate medical terminology.

— Use body maps.

— Use photography in accordance with hospital policy.[12]

1. Consent to photograph may be needed but often is not required by law.

2. Photograph skin against a blue background because white hospital linens reflect light. The use of sterile blue cloths found in hospitals is suggested.

3. Obtain at least 1 photograph with the patient's identification and 1 with a standardized object such as a ruler.

4. Include the time, date, and signature of the photographer and

patient's name and birth date.

5.   If injuries are evolving, document daily.

— Body diagrams, photographs, and handwritten notes must be consistent and accurate.[12]

— Record comments made by family members verbatim.

— Document the identity of persons who provide information.

— If the patient dies before a skeletal survey is obtained, complete the survey before the body leaves the hospital.

PROGNOSIS
— Initial poor prognostic indicators for a child with AHT include unresponsiveness on admission, continued cardiac compromise despite resuscitation efforts, apnea, fixed pupils, no response to pain, DI, severe DIC, or a Glasgow Coma Scale score of 3 to 4.[3]

— Final prognosis may require up to 6 years to become fully realized.[13]

GRIEF AND BEREAVEMENT
— When children die, nursing care continues for families.

1.   The first year of bereavement is associated with increased morbidity and mortality in family members.

2.   Symptoms and conditions such as headaches, fatigue, eating and sleeping disorders, and frequent viral infections are reported.

— The type of grief is unique when children are homicide victims.

1.   Be sensitive to issues.

2.   Prepare parents and other family members for the grieving process.

3.   Rely on hospital chaplain staff members and hospital-based bereavement programs as resources.

4.   Include siblings and grandparents.

5.   Recognize guilt as a significant component when the accused abuser is a family member and nonabusing family members suspected abuse.

6. Understand caregivers may agonize over whether the child suffered.

7. Recognize that homicide can challenge personal spiritual beliefs and cause a loss of trust in society and the criminal justice process.

— Bereavement programs:

1. Address expected issues related to the child's death, but be prepared to handle other issues.

2. Start with phone calls or letters to families from those who worked with them during the hospital stay.

3. Make calls or send cards at intervals throughout the first year, with last contact at or after the anniversary of the child's death.

4. Provide a list of community support groups and educational materials.

5. Provide referrals to victim assistance, victim advocacy programs, and community groups who deal with child homicide.

6. Participate in hospital staff training and counseling from hospital chaplains or social work staff members.[14]

7. Be aware that some institutions make handprints and footprints of the child, gather hospital bracelets and locks of hair, and prepare a memory book in which hospital staff members can write messages to the family or add pictures (with permission).

— Organ donation:

1. Homicide victims can donate organs, but medical staff members must work closely with the police and medical examiner's office for timely coordination of the process.

2. Discuss the issue with law enforcement and medical examiner personnel before presenting it to the family.

EDUCATION
— Educate yourself and the public about child abuse in general and AHT in particular.

— Know the risk factors for abuse and how to identify it quickly.

— Resources include the National Center on Shaken Baby Syndrome (http://www.dontshake.com) and The Shaken Baby Alliance (http://www.shakenbaby.com).

— Attend national conferences focusing on abuse issues.

— Discuss shaken baby syndrome prevention and tips on how to deal with a crying infant with families.

— Provide information on developmental milestones to families of young children so their expectations match their children's abilities.

— Provide information to primary male caregivers.

— Encourage parents to discuss issues with their children's caregivers and to make it clear they are willing to retrieve their children if caregivers get into stressful situations.

REFERENCES

1. Adelson PD, Bratton SL, Carney NA, et al. Guidelines for the acute medical management of severe traumatic brain injury in infants, children, and adolescents. Chapter 4. Resuscitation of blood pressure and oxygenation and prehospital brain-specific therapies for the severe pediatric traumatic brain injury patient. *Pediatr Crit Care Med.* 2003;4(3 suppl):S12-S18.

2. Mazzola CA, Adelson PD. Critical care management of head trauma in children. *Crit Care Med.* 2002;30(11 suppl):S393-S401.

3. Hazinski MF. *Manual of Pediatric Critical Care.* St Louis, Mo: Mosby; 1999.

4. Hymel KP, Abshire TC, Luckey DW, Jenny C. Coagulopathy in pediatric abusive head trauma. *Pediatrics.* 1997;99:371-375.

5. Teasdale G, Jennet B. Assessment of coma and impaired consciousness. A prachcal scale. *Lancet.* 1974;2:81-84.

6. Chiocca EM. Shaken baby syndrome: a nursing perspective. *Pediatr Nurs.* 1995;21:33-38.

7. Hazinski MF. *Nursing Care of the Critically Ill Child*. St Louis, Mo: Mosby; 1992.

8. Adelson PD, Bratton SL, Carney NA, et al. Guidelines for the acute medical management of severe traumatic brain injury in infants, children, and adolescents. Chapter 9. Use of sedation and neuromuscular blockade in the treatment of severe pediatric traumatic brain injury. *Pediatr Crit Care Med*. 2003;4(3 suppl): S34-S37.

9. Arbour R. Using bispectral index monitoring to detect potential breakthrough awareness and limit duration of neuromuscular blockade. *Am J Crit Care*. 2004;13:66-73.

10. Foster JG, Kish SK, Keenan CH. National practice with assessment and monitoring of neuromuscular blockade. *Crit Care Nurs Q*. 2002;25:27-40.

11. Adelson PD, Bratton SL, Carney NA, et al. Guidelines for the acute medical management of severe traumatic brain injury in infants, children, and adolescents. Chapter 18. Nutritional support. *Pediatr Crit Care Med*. 2003;4(3 suppl):S68-S71.

12. Fulton DR. Recognition and documentation of domestic violence in the clinical setting. *Crit Care Nurs Q*. 2000;23:26-34.

13. Conway EE Jr. Nonaccidental head injury in infants: "the shaken baby syndrome revisited." *Pediatr Ann*. 1998;27:677-690.

14. Campbell ML, Thill M. Bereavement follow-up to families after death in the intensive care unit. *Crit Care Med*. 2000;28:1252-1253.

APPENDIX 8-1: CERVICAL SPINE IMMOBILIZATION PROCEDURES

PRINCIPLES

To properly immobilize the cervical spine of pediatric patients requires an appropriately fitted rigid cervical collar and spine board with straps that secure the patient onto the board at the chest, abdomen, and knees (**Appendix Figure 8-1**). Lateral head movement is also restricted using towel rolls and tape or ready-made lateral head stabilizers. Do not obstruct the patient's airway. If the patient's condition allows, build rapport to alleviate the patient's anxiety. Make eye contact, offer comfort measures, and explain procedures in age-appropriate terms. Begin neurological assessment by observing interactions during the primary assessment.

LOGROLLING

First Position

Maintain inline stabilization of the patient's head manually with the straps removed so that the neck is immobilized (**Appendix Figure 8-2**). Position one person at the chest and abdomen and another at the hips and legs. The person at the head controls the roll. Establish clear instructions before rolling so all patient movement can be anticipated. Roll the patient as a single unit into the second position.

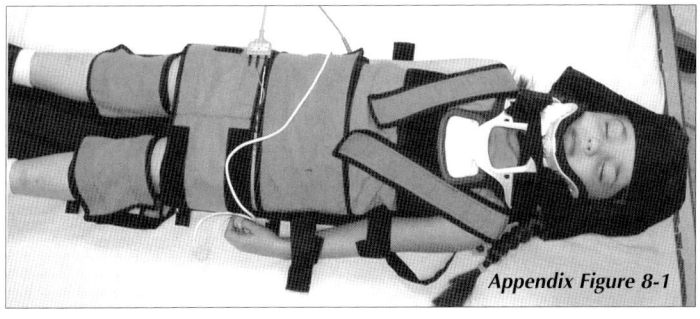

Appendix Figure 8-1

Appendix Figure 8-1. *Proper cervical spine immobilization of the pediatric patient.*

Second Position

This position allows inspection and palpation of the spinal column and posterior surfaces for additional injuries (**Appendix Figure 8-3**). Roll the patient back as a single unit under the direction of the person controlling the head and neck. Maintain manual stabilization until the board straps are reapplied and lateral movement is again restricted.

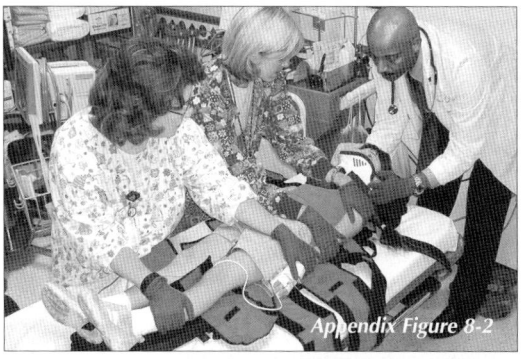

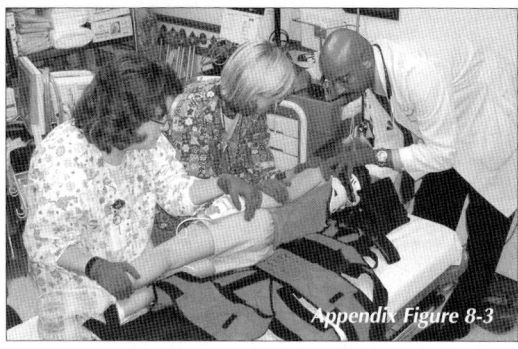

Appendix Figure 8-2. First position of logrolling.

Appendix Figure 8-3. Second position of logrolling.

Photo Credit: *Leslie Pfeil and Michele Rusch*

Participants: *Grace Lett, Laura Lett, RN, Milton Fowler, MD, and Renee Stuckey, RN*

Chapter 9

SOCIAL SERVICES

Wayne I. Munkel, MSW, LCSW
Julie Bradshaw, LCSW

ROLES OF SOCIAL WORKERS

— Help physicians and medical teams obtain details of known history and circumstances of injury.

— Gather information from police and emergency medical personnel and interview parents and/or caregivers.

— Medical social workers serve as liaisons to child protective and law enforcement officers and as coordinators of child protective processes for the hospital.

— Offer tangible support services and emotional support to families of children with abusive head trauma (AHT) who are in crisis.

EVALUATOR

Psychosocial Assessment

— Assessments are recommended as part of a comprehensive team approach.[1-4]

— Assessments give physicians and child protection teams an in-depth analysis of family functioning.

— Begin by focusing on the child.

1. Review the pregnancy, whether it was planned, and how the parents felt about it (**Table 9-1**).

2. Note adjustment to the child's birth (**Table 9-2**).

— Determine other stress factors in the child's home life.

Table 9-1. Pregnancy and Delivery Review Questions

PREGNANCY

— Was the pregnancy planned?

— Did the mother use drugs, alcohol, or tobacco before or during the pregnancy? If so, describe.

— Did the father use drugs, alcohol, or tobacco before or during the pregnancy? If so, describe.

— Describe any emotional stress experienced during the pregnancy.

— Describe any complications experienced during the pregnancy.

DELIVERY

— Was the infant delivered prematurely or full term?

— What was the birth weight of the infant?

— Describe any complications experienced during the delivery.

— Was the infant in the newborn ICU? If so, note length of time and amount of contact with parents.

— Determine whether other children in the family are safe.

1. Note any visible physical signs of abuse and arrange to have a complete physical examination performed by an appropriate medical professional.

2. Determine the children's location, their caregiver, their ages, whether the perpetrator's identity is known, and whether the perpetrator has a history of child or spousal abuse.

3. Maintaining a close working relationship with child protective services (CPS) helps facilitate any necessary physical examinations of siblings.

— Assess the relationship between parental partners.

— Note any history of family violence, poor impulse control, criminal behavior, and drug and alcohol abuse (**Table 9-3**).

Table 9-2. Family's Adjustment to the Infant

FEEDING

— Is the infant nursing?

— Is the infant easy to feed?

— Does the infant have milk allergies or reflux?

— Who feeds the infant? When?

SLEEPING

— Where does the infant sleep? How often? For how many hours?

— Is the infant sleeping through the night?

SOCIAL RESPONSIVENESS

— Is the infant cuddly?

— How does the infant respond to siblings, other caregivers, and when parents or primary caregivers leave?

— How often does the infant cry?

— What do caregivers do when the infant cries?

CHILD'S TEMPERAMENT

— What is the infant's general mood?

— Is the infant adaptable to various situations?

BONDING PROCESS

— Has the family connected with the infant?

— Clarify caregiver responsibilities and how caregivers interact in caring for the children.

— Understand the family dynamic so problems with caring for the child can be anticipated and an appropriate discharge plan can be created.

Developmental Assessment

— Determine expected developmental level of the child before injury.

Table 9-3. Factors Involved in Risk for Child Abuse

— Ages of the parents or caregivers

— Length of parents' or caregivers' relationship (Are they married? Are they living together?)

— Strength of parents' or caregivers' relationship (How often do they argue or disagree?)

— History of family violence, whether current or in family of origin (including child abuse)

— History of drug or alcohol abuse

— History of criminality

— History of depression or mental illness

— History of poor anger management or impulse control

— Current coping strengths and weaknesses

— Job history (Who works? Where and when do they work?)

— Child care (What is each caregiver's role in child care? How much time is spent caring for the child by each caregiver? What type of care is provided?)

— Parenting ability (Are the caregivers knowledgeable about the child's developmental stages? Do they have realistic expectations of the child? Is the child properly supervised?)

— Each parent or caregiver's relationship with the injured child

— Disciplinary practices

— Clarify the child's expected baseline functioning and motor skills, including any disabilities.

— Note phases of childhood especially stressful for caregivers (eg, colic, trained night crying, separation anxiety, exploratory behavior, negativism, poor appetite, and toilet training resistance).[5]

— Determine whether the child is in any of these stages.

History of Injury

— Determining the history of the injury may be the responsibility of medical social workers, child protection team physicians, or CPS and law enforcement officials.

— Use the appropriate investigative model, depending on the regulations of the jurisdiction and the resources available.

— It is difficult to offer emotional support to families after serving in an investigative role, so formal investigative functions are best handled by law enforcement officials, CPS, or both.

— Learn appropriate interviewing techniques in case the medical or social history becomes the primary record of the abusive event.

— Before interviewing parents or caregivers, obtain known medical and social information.

— Note types of injuries and clinical status.

— Ask each parent numerous times to describe how the child was injured.

— Conduct individual interviews with the parents.

— Carefully document stories as part of the medical record, knowing that the record may be subpoenaed for trial.

— Histories explaining the child's injuries may be confusing, false, or not offered at all.[6-8]

— Understand the basics of injury mechanics for determining the validity of information offered by caregivers.

— Determine when the child was last acting normally.

— Determine who was caring for the child at the time of injury.

— Create a timeline and clarify the sequence of events preceding the injury.

— Prepare and compare timelines with law enforcement officials and child protection investigators to confirm or contradict histories and clarify time and place of injury.

— When parents describe falls as the cause of injury, document the details of the fall (eg, distance fallen, surface on which the child landed, and the condition and behavior of the child when found).

— Work with law enforcement and child protection investigators to determine whether the location and circumstances are accurate as described.[9,10]

— With the medical team, prosecutors, the guardian *ad litem*, law enforcement officials, and CPS all present, discuss the case from every angle.

1. The medical team clarifies misunderstandings about complex terms or findings.

2. Law enforcement officials and CPS explain crime scene details.

3. Review timeline of events.

4. Identify missing pieces and make appropriate assignments.

5. Prosecutors and the guardian *ad litem* make an informed decision about whether the case should go to court.

COORDINATOR

— The role is primarily one of connecting various hospital team members with outside agencies and helping all to obtain necessary information about the abused child.

— Begins as soon as the decision to refer to CPS is made.

— Prepare reports on injuries, why nonaccidental causes are suspected, the child's and parents' demographic and contact information, and any relevant history.

— Once the report is prepared, serve as liaison with CPS, law enforcement, and court officials.

1. Facilitate information flow about children and their safety between hospital and protective agencies.

2. If children are placed in protective custody by the court and the parents are denied visitation, relay this information to charge nurses and make certain it is written prominently in the medical record.

3. If other children are at risk, quickly relay information to CPS so protective steps can be taken.

4. Assist individuals from outside agencies with meeting each new medical care team and negotiating each new part of the medical system.

5. As children's cases move through the juvenile justice and child welfare systems, CPS case workers are sometimes replaced by foster care workers. Introduce new members to medical care teams, hospital processes, and family members.

— Offer supportive services.

1. Include pastoral care, mental health services, and family support services.

2. Because children with severe head injuries require days to weeks of treatment and care, most parents want to stay with the child. Petition hospitals to provide lodging, food, and transportation assistance.

3. Arrange for financial assistance during hospitalization.

— Care for medical staff members in the emergency department and intensive care unit.

1. These persons are particularly prone to secondary trauma because of constant, long-term exposure to traumatic events.

2. Critical incident stress-management teams help staff members address their own traumatic stress issues when AHT results in a child homicide or extremely critical injuries.

3. Recognize which staff members need professional assistance from therapists or employee assistance programs.

— Assist with rehabilitation services.

1. Most children with severe head injuries do not return to baseline functioning. Prepare the family for this possibility and for long-term health care needs.

2. Participate in decisions regarding institutional care, complex home health care, and referrals to specialists after discharge or in the future.

— Be involved in discharge planning.

1. Prepare caregivers to meet children's medical, social, psychological, and spiritual needs.

2. Coordinate the flow of information to and from physicians, nurses, therapists, and other hospital staff members associated with ongoing care and treatment of abused children to ensure a smooth transition from hospital to community.

— Regarding the death of a child:

1. Realize that death from AHT can occur after hours, days, or weeks.

2. Work with the hospital's pastoral care staff and other hospital staff members to help parents prepare for the death.

3. Help with funeral plans.

4. Help with the issue of organ donation, coordinating communication among the local transplant agency, medical examiner or coroner, and parents.

FATALITY REVIEW, PREVENTION, AND ADVOCACY
— Death from AHT is eligible for review in states with fatality review programs.

1. Examine child abuse deaths to prevent future deaths and address problems with CPS processes.

2. Produce data on child abuse deaths and suggest ways to prevent them.

— Represent the hospital or arrange for hospital representatives to be at review meetings.

REFERENCES
1. Freitag R, Lazoritz S, Kini N. Psychosocial aspects of child abuse for primary care pediatricians. *Pediatr Clin North Am.* 1998;45: 391-402.

2. Krugman RD, Bays JA, Chadwick DL, Kanda M, Levitt C, McHugh MT, for the American Academy of Pediatrics. Committee

on Child Abuse and Neglect. Shaken baby syndrome: inflicted cerebral trauma. *Pediatrics*. 1993;92:872-875.

3. Morris MW, Smith S, Cressman J, Ancheta J. Evaluation of infants with subdural hematoma who lack external evidence of abuse. *Pediatrics*. 2000;105:549-553.

4. Quayle K. Minor head injury in the pediatric patient. *Pediatr Clin North Am*. 1999;46:1189-1199.

5. Schmitt BD. Seven deadly sins of childhood: advising parents about difficult developmental phases. *Child Abuse Negl*. 1987;11: 421-432.

6. Chadwick DL, Chin S, Salerna C, Landsverk J, Kitchen L. Deaths from falls in children: how far is fatal? *J Trauma*. 1991;31:1353-1355.

7. Duhaime AC, Christian CW, Rorke LB, Zimmerman RA. Nonaccidental head injury in infants—the "shaken-baby syndrome." *N Engl J Med*. 1998;338:1823-1829.

8. Reece RM, Sege R. Childhood head injuries: accidental or inflicted? *Arch Pediatr Adolesc Med*. 2000;154:11-15.

9. Conway EE. Nonaccidental head injury in infants: "the shaken baby syndrome revisited." *Pediatr Ann*. 1998;27:677-690.

10. Wilkins B. Head injury—abuse or accident? *Arch Dis Child*. 1997;76:393-397.

Chapter 10

AUTOPSY FINDINGS

Sam P. Gulino, MD

Gregory A. Schmunk, MD, FACP, FASCP

CHILD DEATH INVESTIGATION

— Deaths caused by violent injury (suicide, homicide, or accident) are reportable to the medical examiner or coroner.

— Investigation requires cooperation between the medical examiner or coroner, police, and child protective services (CPS).

1. The medical examiner or coroner identifies the cause and manner of death.

   A. *Medical examiner*. Usually a physician, typically a forensic pathologist, appointed to serve at the state or county level.

   B. *Coroner*. Elected position held by any person eligible to run for office. Nonphysician coroners typically contract with pathologists for autopsy services.

2. Police investigate evidence of a crime for purposes of criminal prosecution (see Chapter 11, Forensic Investigations).

3. The safety of other children in the household is of interest to CPS.

— Each agency must share information with others and maintain good relationships with medical caregivers.

FORENSIC PATHOLOGISTS

— May be the only medical professionals in a community with specific training to differentiate abusive from accidental injuries and recognize patterned injuries.

— May be a resource in evaluating living children, both when they may die and when they are expected to survive.

— Coordinate efforts in complex cases requiring multidisciplinary approach.

— Are, most importantly, objective observers of facts without regard for whether they aid the prosecution or defense in a criminal case or the plaintiff or defendant in a civil case.

— Require complete information on the subject's medical history, the family's social history, the circumstances of the injury, and prehospital and hospital medical care.

1. Hypotheses are based on initial investigative information and are modified by the results of the autopsy, ancillary studies, and additional data.

2. Unexplained findings prompt further investigation and may prompt additional postmortem studies.

3. Pathologists anticipate questions and collect data to formulate answers.

— Use and/or contribute to factual case data, including medical records, witness interviews, scene investigations, and autopsy findings.

1. Record data by whatever means are appropriate.

2. Express descriptions in neutral language.

— Determine the cause and manner of death and, when trauma is found, the timing, mechanism, and lethality of injuries.

— Death certification:

1. Certifier is required to opine on the disease process, injury, or combination that led to death (*cause of death*) as well as the ***manner of death***, which is a one-word opinion of the circumstances in which death occurred.

    A. *Natural.* Only when the person died of a natural disease; trauma plays no role.

B. *Accidental*. Death caused by an unintentional event, even when preventable.

C. *Suicide*. Person showed intent to cause self-harm either explicitly or implicitly.

D. *Homicide*. Death is a direct result of the action of at least one person against another. It is not necessary to show intent to kill or harm. The medicolegal concept is separate from the legal concepts of homicide, murder, and manslaughter. Does not imply that someone is criminally culpable.

E. *Undetermined*. Death is clearly not natural but cannot be ascertained as an accident, suicide, or homicide.

— Express opinions verbally, in correspondence, in deposition, or at trial.

— Draw conclusions with a "reasonable degree of medical certainty," which is presumably based on an accepted body of medical knowledge.

PROCEDURES BEFORE AUTOPSY

— With adequate preliminary investigative data, scene investigation, and medical history, pathologists can:

1. Plan special procedures before or during the autopsy.

2. Ensure the autopsy is geared toward answering questions that arise.

3. Interpret injuries, artifacts, and signs of medical intervention in context.

4. Evaluate the mechanism, timing, and lethality of injuries.

— Review preliminary medical and investigative history and communicate directly with treating physicians.

— Scene investigation:

1. Assess the environment to identify mechanisms of specific injuries.

2. Death scene reviews are done by police agency, crime scene investigation unit, or the medical examiner/coroner. Leaders of agencies must clarify responsibilities to ensure a thorough investigation.

— Technically, pathologists can perform autopsies with no advance information.

1. The autopsy is limited to a list of findings without evaluating significance.

2. Pathologists cannot anticipate the need for special procedures.

TRACE EVIDENCE RECOVERY

— Police typically determine whether trace evidence recovery is needed.

— Police, a criminalist, a pathologist, or a combination may collect such evidence.

— Handle the body as little as possible before evidence collection to prevent evidence loss or contamination.

— If a body must be moved before evidence collection:

1. Wrap the body in a clean sheet.

2. After unwrapping it, submit the sheet for trace evidence analysis.

— The 2 categories of evidence recovery are:

1. Hair and fiber recovery.

2. Evidence of sexual assault.

— Procedure for hair and fiber collection:

1. Carefully inspect clothing and skin surface visually under adequate lighting and with a handheld magnifier.

2. Remove hair and fibers with forceps and place into appropriate containers. The crime laboratory assessing the evidence determines the appropriate packaging.

3. Maintain a rigorous chain of custody.

— Procedure for sexual assault evidence collection:

1. Evidence is collected when injuries to genitalia or perineum are seen or there is historical or circumstantial evidence suggesting sexual assault.

2. Ready-made kits:

    A. Are usually designed for adults and may not be appropriate for children.

    B. Include:

      (1) Preliminary documentation of the genitalia and anus.

      (2) Serologic and DNA evidence obtained by swabbing the oral cavity, anus, and vagina (or perineum and vaginal vestibule in prepubertal girls, if the hymen is normal).

    C. In male victims, swab penile skin using swabs moistened with sterile saline solution in addition to the oral cavity and anus.

    D. Place smears on glass slides to identify sperm.

    E. Collect possible seminal fluid on skin surfaces.

3. Collect evidence before washing the body.

4. Using a vaginal speculum and anoscope to recover specimens from the vagina and anus may be helpful.

    A. Document the presence or absence of injuries to the hymen and anus and photograph both before using these devices.

    B. Consider the size of the child when choosing instruments.

— Alternative light sources:

1. Vary from handheld flashlights with Wood's filters to large plug-in units with variable wavelength adapters.

2. Various wavelengths enhance certain fibers and body fluids, so they can be identified, photographed with filters, and collected.

POSTMORTEM RADIOGRAPHY

— Include a skeletal evaluation in all cases of suspected abuse.

— Simple anteroposterior (AP) radiographs that identify skeletal trauma in infants are not sufficient in suspected abuse cases.

— High-detail skeletal surveys identify subtle acute and healing metaphyseal and rib fractures[1,2] and should be obtained in all cases of suspected abuse.

— Factors affecting the ability to obtain a full skeletal survey:

1. Circumstances surrounding death

2. Budget

3. Availability of a technician able to perform skeletal surveys

— Postmortem magnetic resonance imaging:

1. May identify lesions before autopsy and guide brain evaluation.[3]

2. Has no clear role in evaluating abusive head trauma (AHT).

— Is not useful for lesions of the upper cervical spinal cord.[4]

— Autopsy is still standard for identifying intracranial hemorrhages, particularly small interhemispheric subdural hematomas.

CONDUCTING THE AUTOPSY

— The autopsy is a tool to evaluate how death occurred (**Figure 10-1**).

— Statutes do not usually specify when autopsies are required, leaving the decision to the medical examiner/coroner.

Figure 10-1.
Concept of the autopsy in a poorly designed death investigation system. The pathologist is provided with little or no information and is expected to draw conclusions.

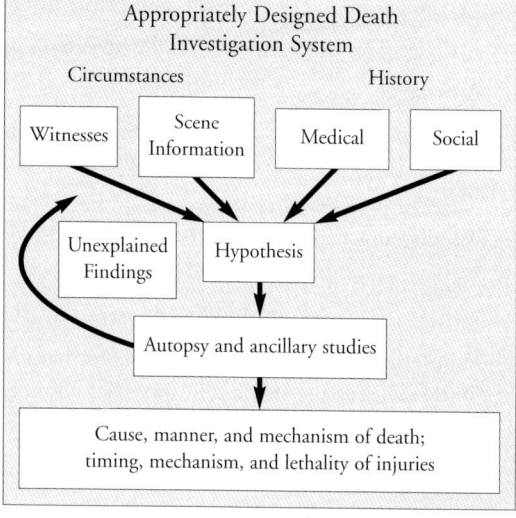

Appropriately Designed Death Investigation System

Circumstances   History

Witnesses | Scene Information | Medical | Social

Unexplained Findings | Hypothesis

Autopsy and ancillary studies

Cause, manner, and mechanism of death; timing, mechanism, and lethality of injuries

— Cases requiring autopsy vary by local custom, philosophy of practice, and needs of the police and prosecutors.

— Autopsy is indicated in all cases of AHT.

— Ideally, all infants and small children with head injuries are autopsied.

1. Standard for identifying and describing injuries:

    A. Autopsy can discover injuries that are not apparent clinically or radiographically.

    B. The nature, extent, and age of injury are better defined by postmortem examination.

2. Autopsies allow for better differentiation between abusive and nonabusive head injury.

3. Findings accompanying AHT can include thoracoabdominal or other, less visible injuries.

— Generally, the medical examiner/coroner can perform an autopsy without permission from next of kin and despite objections from the family.

1. The best approach is to educate the family about the procedure and purpose of the autopsy.

2. Include the family or community religious leader in the discussion.

3. Know about special procedures that make autopsy more acceptable.

EXTERNAL FINDINGS

— Describe any items, including clothing and diapers, received with the body.

— Note the apparent state of development, nutrition, and hydration.

1. Note the general state of hygiene before the body is washed.

2. Note the presence and degree of postmortem changes.

3. Measure height (length), weight, head circumference, and chest circumference and plot on growth charts as objective proof of development and nutrition.

4. Describe individual identifying features.

— Systematically describe external aspects of the body from head to toe.

— Document the absence of specific findings as *pertinent negatives.*

1. Include the absence of conjunctival petechiae; scleral discoloration; injuries to oral mucosa, genitalia, and anus; and internal injuries not reflected by visible skin injuries.

2. Note medical interventions to avoid confusion with injuries.

3. Standard autopsy diagrams show the relative location of injury on the body surface.

— Photography:

1. Permits objective assessment, free of subjective alterations.

2. Subtle findings indistinct to the naked eye may become obvious when a photograph is enlarged or a transparency is projected on a screen.

3. Use liberally at multiple magnification levels.

4. Include an L-shaped ruler when photographing patterned injuries.

5. Compare dental casts or objects with photographed injuries.

— Tracing injury onto transparent material:

1. Preserves the configuration of patterned injury.

2. Compare putative weapons with tracing.

3. Is useful during the period after the body is released, before autopsy photographs are available.

— Sample cutaneous wounds.

1. Excise for histologic examination.

2. Group injuries into distinct age groups.[5,6]

3. Determine the minimum number of traumatic episodes.

Bite Marks
— Before the body is washed, swab the skin surface from the central

portion of the bite mark with a moistened swab to collect saliva for serologic and DNA analysis.

— A forensic odontologist may advocate removing the skin bearing the bite mark for preservation or creating molded impressions of bite marks.[7]

INTERNAL EXAMINATION

— After opening the thoracoabdominal cavity through a Y-shaped incision, document the presence of blood or other abnormal fluid collections in body cavities.

1. Collect the blood into a graduated measuring container and note volume.

2. Photograph the container for added documentation.

— During evisceration, collect specimens for toxicological testing.

1. The types and packaging of specimens are usually dictated by the laboratory that performs the testing.

2. Collect specimens to exclude the presence of natural diseases.

3. Cultures of blood, spleen, lung, spinal fluid, etc, rule out or diagnose infection.

— Tests for inborn errors of metabolism:

1. Are done using spots of dried blood or bile on filter paper, similar to newborn screening cards.

2. Should be routinely included in infant and child autopsies.

3. May reveal abnormalities affecting other children in the family.

— After evisceration, weigh and examine the organs.

1. Evaluate for the presence or absence of injury or natural disease.

2. Take tissue samples for histologic examination.

— Examine vertebral bodies and ribs for healed and recent fractures.

1. Excise, decalcifiy, and examine histologically those identified on preautopsy radiographs and at autopsy.

2. For ribs, follow histologic criteria for the aging of fractures.

3. For other fractures, classify as acute, healing, or healed.

4. When multiple rib fractures are present, resect the complete rib cage and take additional radiographs as needed.

5. Alternatively, create radiographs of resected rib cages with a mammography machine using multiple projections. The resulting films are highly detailed and magnified.

SPECIAL TECHNIQUES FOR EXAMINATION OF THE HEAD AND NECK

— Document, diagram, and photograph external injuries to the scalp and face.

— Shave hair so injuries in hair-bearing portions of the scalp can be clearly seen.

— Examine subcutaneous tissues for hemorrhage.

— Incise and reflect temporalis muscles for hemorrhages.

— Document injuries to the scalp and temporalis muscles photographically.

— When no impact injuries are visible on the skin surface, deep scalp, or temporalis muscles, take photographs showing this pertinent negative finding.

— Subgaleal hemorrhage is produced by impact and is located in the potential space between the galea aponeurotica and the skull (**Figures 10-2-a** and **b**). It is often seen when impact is associated with underlying calvarial fracture.

1. Remove the galea and reflect temporalis muscles to document the presence or absence of calvarial vault fractures.

2. Describe fractures by size, location, shape (linear, branching, stellate, comminuted), and depth of bony fragment depression (if seen).

3. Photograph or diagram all vault fractures before opening the head.

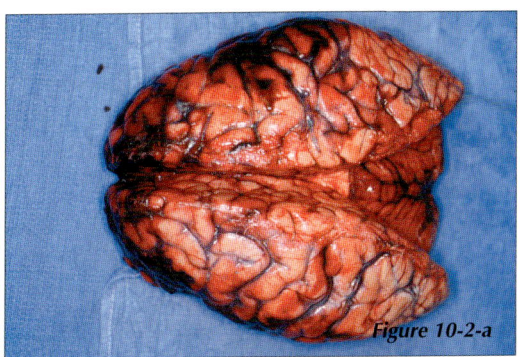

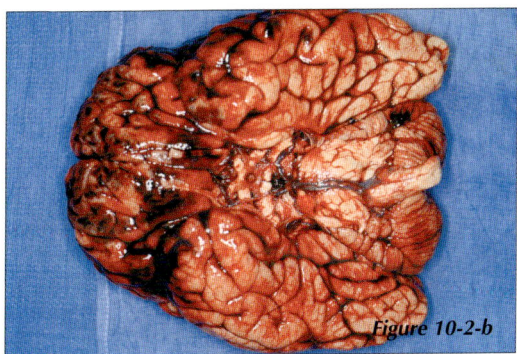

Figures 10-2-a and **b.** *The brain of this man, who was found on an ice-covered driveway, has extensive contrecoup contusions of the frontal and anterior temporal lobes of the brain. Such injuries are rarely seen in infant head injury but are common in adults.*

4. Open the calvaria using an oscillating autopsy saw. Do not cut into the brain parenchyma.

   A. This procedure is more difficult when the child has survived long enough to develop significant cerebral edema (**Figures 10-3-a** and **b**).

   B. Dural connections to the falx cerebri and tentorium cerebelli often remain intact after sawing.

195

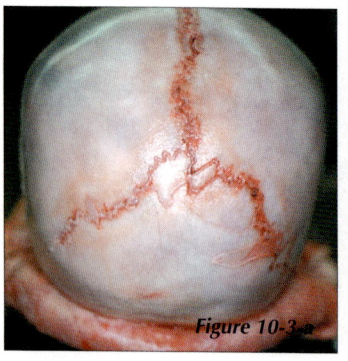
Figure 10-3-a

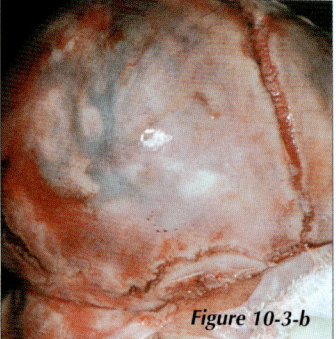
Figure 10-3-b

Figures 10-3-a and b. Diastasis of cranial sutures indicate severe cerebral edema.

    C. If needed, incise with a scalpel before removing the calvarial cap.

5.   Remove the brain carefully; minimize postmortem artifact.

    A. Infant brains are typically very soft because of high water content. They are especially soft when children are resuscitated and maintained on ventilators.

    B. Do not examine an infant's brain immediately; fix it in 10% buffered formalin solution for 10 to 14 days before sectioning.

    C. Section the brain in consultation with a neuropathologist experienced in interpreting brain injuries in infants and children.

— Subdural hemorrhage (**Figures 10-4-a** and **b**):

1.   Often adheres to the dura mater, though adherence of fresh hemorrhages may be minimal.

2.   Document photographically, and then strip the dura mater from the inner table of the calvaria and skull base, keeping the subdural hemorrhage intact and adherent when possible.

— Removing the dura mater reveals epidural hemorrhages, often associated with overlying skull fracture and skull base fractures.

— Take samples of the dura mater and adherent hematoma for histologic testing.

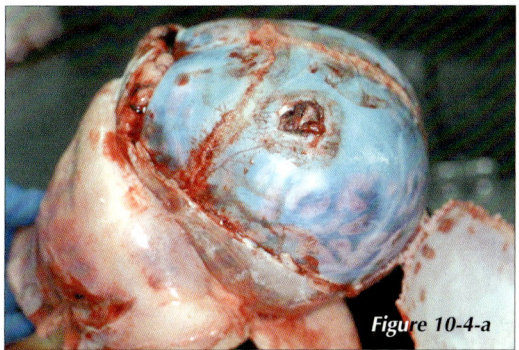

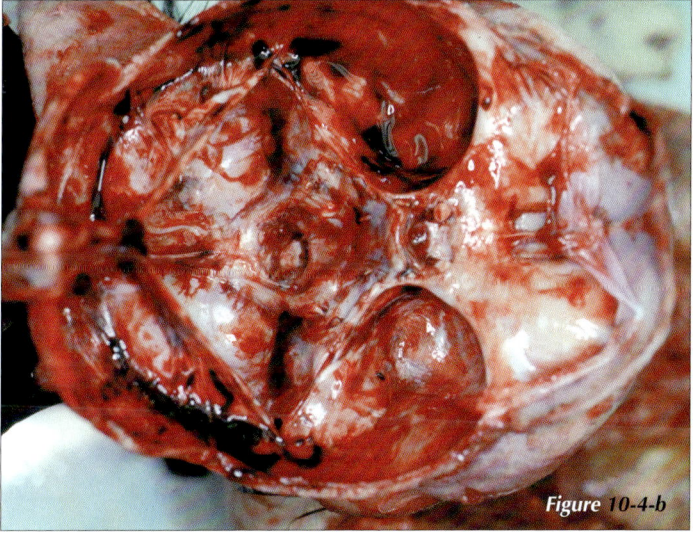

Figure 10-4-a. Subdural hematoma beneath the tense dura mater. The central hemorrhagic area represents the site of an emergent craniotomy to relieve elevated intracranial pressure. This dura mater had completely separated from the overlying bone during swelling of the brain.

Figure 10-4-b. Base of skull demonstrating subdural hematoma once the brain is removed.

1. Determine the age of the hematoma by noting if it is free of organization, in early or late stages of organization, or organized.

2. Take sections of bone along the edges of skull fractures to demonstrate healing.

3. Infer age of skull fractures from gross appearance and associated injuries.

Examination of the Neck by Posterior Approach

— Dissect the posterior neck in all AHT cases. Forces that injure the brain can affect the cervical spine and its ligaments or injure the spinal cord.

— Dissect the posterior cervical and suboccipital muscles layer by layer, noting any intramuscular hemorrhages.

1. Examine the spinous process for fractures.

2. Remove posterior elements of the cervical spine to expose the spinal cord, noting hemorrhages.

3. Inspect posterior longitudinal ligaments, transverse ligaments, alar ligaments, the tectorial membrane, atlanto-occipital joints, and atlantoaxial joints for strains and lacerations.

4. Retain the spinal cord and brain for assessment after formalin fixation.

Examination of Vertebral Arteries

— Suspect injury to vertebral arteries based on clinical or radiographic evidence of vertebrobasilar ischemia or unexplained basilar subarachnoid hemorrhage.

1. Examine radiographically and by direct inspection after the brain is removed.

2. Cannulate arteries at their origins from the subclavian arteries.

3. Depending on an infant's size, inject 1 to 5 mL of water-soluble contrast material and take AP radiographs immediately.

    A. Complete arterial lacerations appear as foci of contrast extravasation.

   B. Vertebral artery dissection appears as segmental narrowing of the lumen.

— After dissecting the cervical spine, paraspinal musculature, and cervical spinal cord, inspect arteries directly.

1. Remove the posterior laminae and posterior portions of transverse processes, using an oscillating saw to unroof channels where arteries lie.

2. Note frank blood extravasation with complete laceration or hemorrhagic discoloration of arterial adventitia with arterial dissection.

Eye Dissection

— Remove the eyes via posterior, intracranial approach.

1. Inspect orbital roofs for fractures, then remove orbital roofs using an oscillating saw.

2. Remove canal roofs for optic nerves.

3. Examine orbital contents, noting hemorrhages in orbital fat or extraocular muscles and preserving maximum length of optic nerve (**Figure 10-5**).

— Delay sectioning to permit 4 to 5 days of formalin fixation.

1. Note hemorrhage in optic nerve sheaths externally.

2. Transect optic nerves 4 to 5 mm from globes and embed them in cross section for histologic examination (**Figure 10-6**).

— Dissect eyes.

1. Open the eyes using a horizontal cut, bisecting each eye along its AP axis, using posterior ciliary vessels to indicate the horizontal eye axis.

2. Examine the interior of each globe half for retinal hemorrhages and photograph them.

3. Can place another horizontal section parallel to the first to obtain a specimen suitable for embedding for histologic examination (**Figure 10-7**).

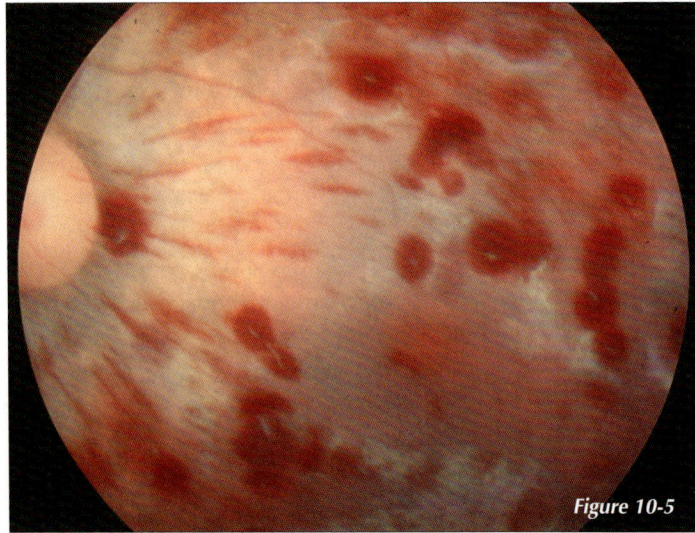

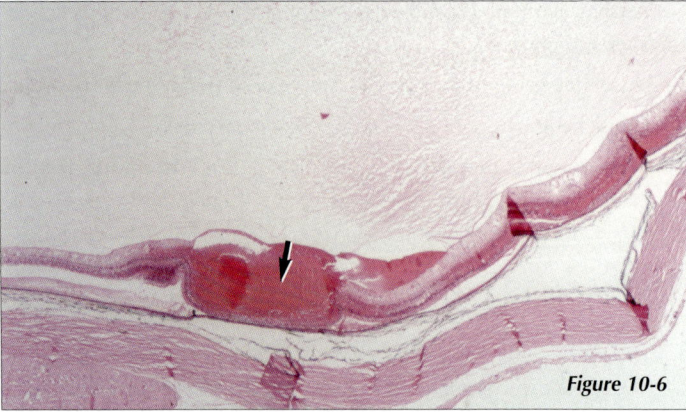

Figure 10-5. *White-centered retinal hemorrhages that are confined to the posterior pole.*

Figure 10-6. *Photomicrograph of specimen of the retina demonstrating extensive retinal hemorrhages (arrow), which were seen in representative sections in both eyes extending to the periphery.*

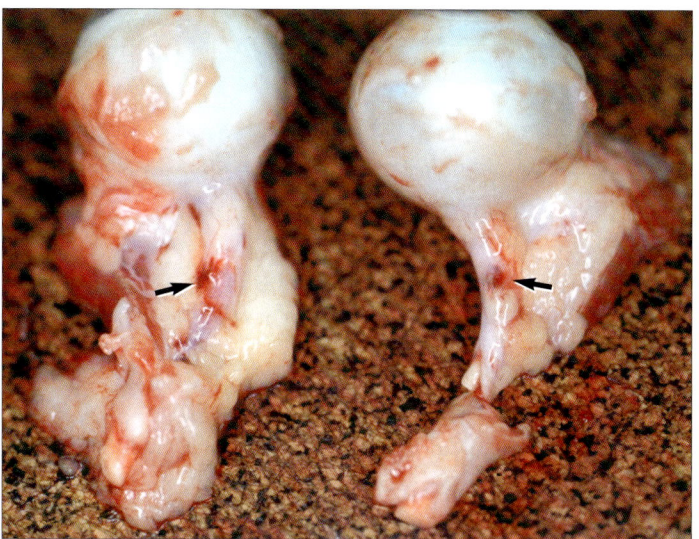

Figure 10-7. Bilateral optic nerve sheath hemorrhages (arrows).

— In hospitalized children who have had indirect ophthalmoscopy, section the eye to simulate the appearance during fundoscopic examination.

1. Make a single coronal cut immediately posterior to the ciliary body, removing the cornea, anterior chamber, lens, and iris.

2. Look directly into the cup-shaped globe, simulating a clinical eye examination.

3. If histologic sections are needed, make an AP cut also.

— With suspected head injury and dehydration or malnutrition, collect the vitreous humor to determine electrolyte levels.

1. Slowly withdraw vitreous fluid from 1 eye using a small-gauge needle (22 gauge) and submit the fluid for studies.

2. Reinflate the globe by injecting 10% formalin solution in the same volume as the withdrawn fluid.

3. Fix the eye in formalin and examine it.

4. Perform on only one eye so the other eye can be examined free of artifact.

NOTE: This procedure may produce artifactual retinal detachment but does not cause artifactual hemorrhage if performed carefully and slowly.

AUTOPSY FINDINGS IN AHT

CONTACT INJURIES

— Are caused by directly striking the head with an object or by impact of the head with a surface. They are usually located directly under the site of impact.

— Scalp contusions, abrasions, and lacerations are seen with blunt injury, but children and infants may have little externally apparent scalp injury even with significant impact (**Figures 10-8-a** and **b**).

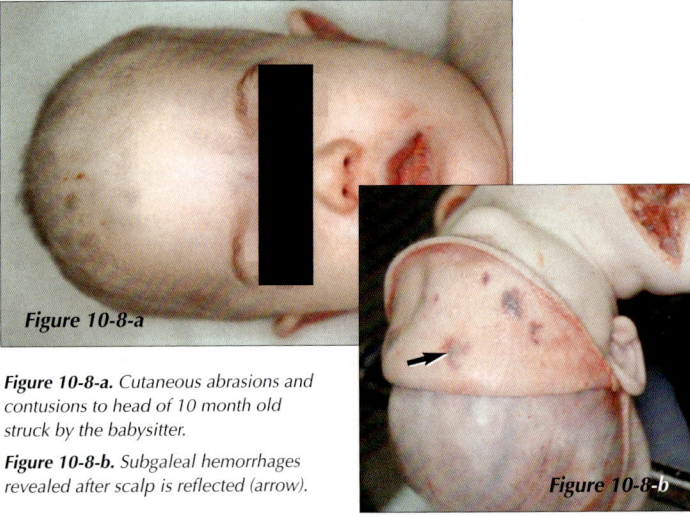

Figure 10-8-a.

Figure 10-8-a. Cutaneous abrasions and contusions to head of 10 month old struck by the babysitter.

Figure 10-8-b. Subgaleal hemorrhages revealed after scalp is reflected (arrow).

Figure 10-8-b

1. Impact sites are often visible after reflecting the scalp, as hemorrhages in subcutaneous soft tissues may not extend to the skin surface.

2. Even when no injuries are seen at autopsy, impact may have occurred.[8]

3. Visible contusions provide the minimum number of impacts. The maximum number is not determinable.

— Skull fractures occur when pressure on the skull at the impact site exceeds bone tolerance.

1. Skull fractures are seen under impact sites in accidental and abusive head injuries. Linear fractures are possible in both groups.

2. Complex, depressed, and multiple fractures are more common in abuse or automobile crashes.[9,10]

3. Skull fractures are also seen with blood collections between the external aspect of the skull and the galea aponeurotica (subgaleal hematoma) (**Figures 10-9-a** and **b**).

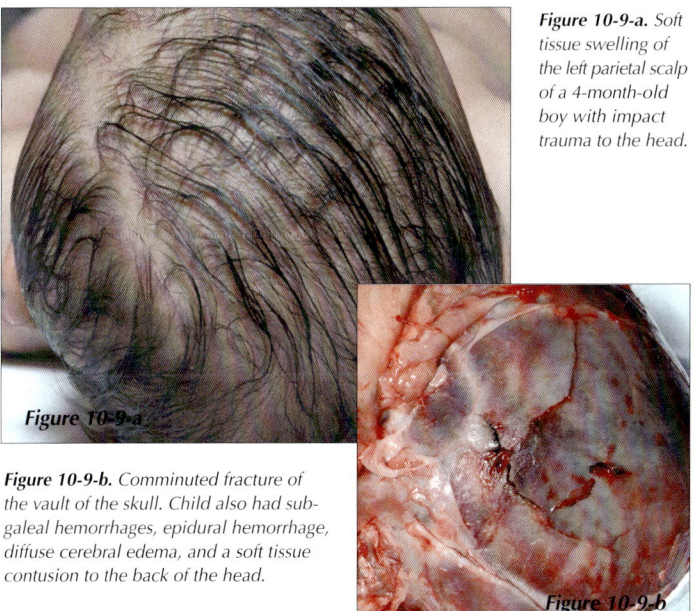

Figure 10-9-a. *Soft tissue swelling of the left parietal scalp of a 4-month-old boy with impact trauma to the head.*

Figure 10-9-a

Figure 10-9-b. *Comminuted fracture of the vault of the skull. Child also had subgaleal hemorrhages, epidural hemorrhage, diffuse cerebral edema, and a soft tissue contusion to the back of the head.*

Figure 10-9-b

— Epidural hematoma:

1. Is common when the artery is torn as the overlying skull is fractured; however, in children, most are not accompanied by skull fracture.[11]

2. The artery tears as the skull bends during impact, then rebounds sharply (**Figure 10-10**).

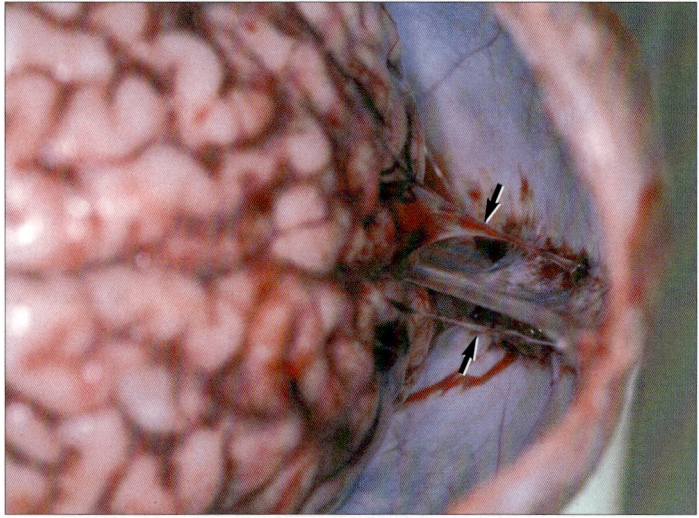

Figure 10-10. *Intact bridging veins at autopsy (arrows).*

— *Coup contusions* are cerebral cortical contusions at the site of impact resulting from direct transmission of force to the brain.

— *Contrecoup contusions* are cerebral cortical contusions opposite the site of impact resulting from skull volume changes and motion of the brain in the skull.[12]

1. They are common in adults with head trauma and help distinguish injuries incurred in a fall (predominantly contrecoup) from those caused by a blow to the head (predominantly coup).

2. They are seldom seen in infants and small children.[13]

— Avoid improper use of the 2 previous terms.

INERTIAL INJURIES

— ***Impact loading*** results from head motion and is induced by striking the head and causing it to move.

— ***Impulsive loading*** or ***whiplash*** occurs when the head is induced to move without direct impact.

Subdural Hematoma

— Results when bridging veins tear due to the brain moving within the calvarial vault.

— Is probably present in most cases of clinically significant inertial head injury[14] but missed on clinical imaging.[15]

— Must remove the calvaria after it is sawed so small subdural hemorrhages are not missed and blood draining artifactually from incised dural sinuses is not confused with antemortem subdural hemorrhage.

Diffuse Axonal Injury

— Has important implications for timing injuries.

— Subdural hematomas, especially when thin and bilateral, are markers for inertial head motion and indicate conditions in which traumatic axonal injury occurs.[16]

— The pathologic diagnosis of traumatic diffuse axonal injury requires axonal damage to be diffuse and traumatic, or mechanical, in origin.

1. Occurs in the centrum semiovale, corpus callosum, and other large white matter bundles.[17]

2. Need an adequate sample for histologic diagnosis.[18]

— Distinguish between traumatic axonal injury and axonal injury related to hypoxia or at the edges of infarcted brain.

— Diagnose using standard hematoxylin-eosin stains and silver stains to identify axonal retraction bulbs (axonal accumulation bulbs).

1. Methods lack sensitivity to detect axonal injury 18 to 24 hours after injury.

2. Immunohistochemical staining for beta-amyloid precursor protein enhances results.[18-21]

3. Damaged axons found about 2 hours after injury; foci of axonal accumulation are visible about 3 hours postinjury.[19]

— Tissue tear hemorrhages or contusional tears are rare.[16,22]

1. They are usually seen at the interface between the cortex and subcortical white matter.

2. They result from differential motion of portions of the brain with different densities during head motion.

INJURIES AT THE CRANIOCERVICAL JUNCTION

— These injuries are components of battered child syndrome.[23-27]

— Differentiate artifactual discharge of blood from epidural venous plexus from antemortem hemorrhage.

— Findings in the spinal cord and brainstem (**Figures 10-11-a, b, c, and d**), not extra-axial hemorrhages, guide interpretation.

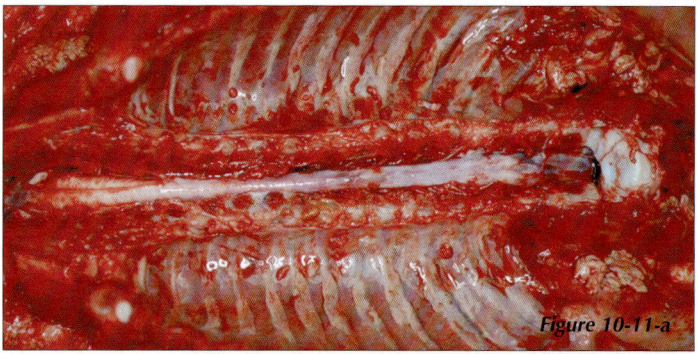

Figure 10-11-a

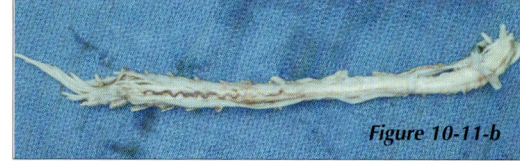

*Figures 10-11-a and **b**. Spinal cord, in situ (a) and after removal and fixation (b), showing no evidence of injury.*

Figure 10-11-b

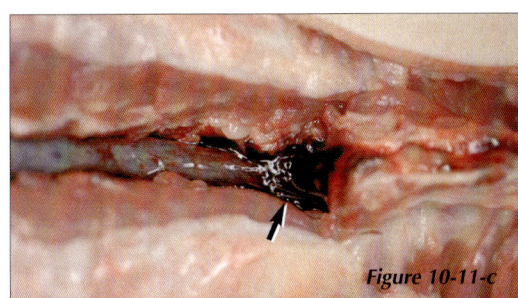

Figures 10-11-c
*and **d**. Epidural
and subdural
hemorrhages of the
cervical and lum-
bar spinal cord
without a history
of spinal tap
(arrows).*

Figure 10-11-c

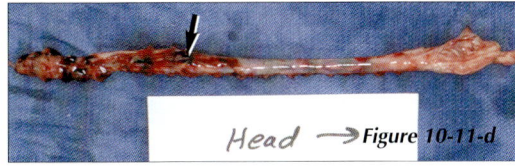

Figure 10-11-d

SECONDARY BRAIN CHANGES

Hypoxia and Ischemia

— May result from increased intracranial pressure, occlusion of cerebral vessels during herniation, systemic hypotension, and respiratory depression or apnea causing global hypoxemia.[28,29]

— May find evidence of early diffuse hypoxic-ischemic injury in hippocampal neurons and cerebellar Purkinje cells.[29]

— In long-term survivors, the brain may have widespread pseudo-laminar necrosis of the cortex and rarefaction of white matter, changes that obscure original injuries.

Cerebral Edema

— The term is not diagnostically helpful without explaining the underlying cause.

— In AHT, cerebral edema may result from trauma such as traumatic axonal injury, diffuse hypoxic-ischemic injury caused by hypotension and/or apnea, changes in cerebral blood flow and vascular permea-bility, or metabolic derangement.[16,29]

— Examine the brain and review medical history to distinguish hypoxic from traumatic axonal injury.

1. Initial neurologic symptoms and degree of lucidity directly reflect primary brain injury.

2. Subsequent neurologic deterioration reflects sequelae (**Figure 10-12**).

3. Cerebral edema is not a reliable indicator of time since injury.[30]

Eye Pathology

— Finding multiple hemorrhages diffusely in both eyes raises possibility of abusive inertial head injury, but not all infants with such injuries have retinal hemorrhages[31] (**Figure 10-13**).

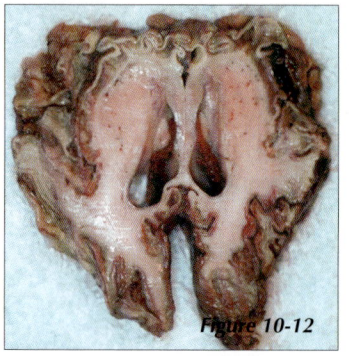 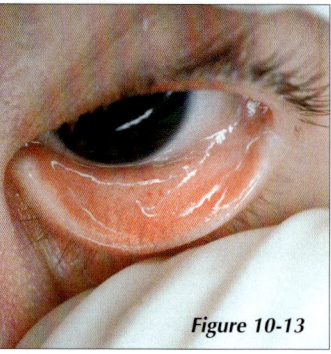

Figure 10-12. *Coronal section of brain of 3-month-old girl shaken 2 months prior to her death. Bilateral organized subdural membranes and extensive encephalomalacia as revealed during autopsy.*

Figure 10-13. *Focal ocular petechiae, which are consistent with resuscitative efforts. Thymic petechiae were also present (not shown).*

— Retinal hemorrhages occur in infants and children with severe accidental head injuries, but the hemorrhages are typically less severe, unilateral, and confined to the posterior pole of the eye.[32-34]

— There is no support for cardiopulmonary resuscitation as a cause.

— Retinoschisis and retinal detachment are seen in abusive inertial head injury[31] and are purely mechanical or traumatic in origin.

— Hemorrhage in the optic nerve sheath is often seen in abusive inertial head injury.[31]

ORGAN AND TISSUE DONATION

VASCULAR ORGAN DONATION

— The medical examiner/coroner usually reviews cases of potential donors and approves donation.

— The body is examined and photographed before anything is taken for donation so that surgical artifact is not confused with antemortem injury.

— Appropriate diagnostic studies are required to document normal function and absence of injury in viscera that will be disrupted or removed during organ retrieval.

POSTMORTEM TISSUE DONATION

— Does not share the same urgency or necessity as vascular organ donation.

— Infants and children usually only qualify as donors of heart valves and corneas.

REFERENCES

1. Kleinman PK, Marks SC Jr, Richmond JM, Blackbourne BD. Inflicted skeletal injury: a postmortem radiologic-histopathologic study in 31 infants. *AJR Am J Roentgenol*. 1995;165:647-650.

2. Kleinman PK, Marks SC Jr, Nimkin K, Rayder SM, Kessler SC. Rib fractures in 31 abused infants: postmortem radiologic-histopathologic study. *Radiology*. 1996;200:807-810.

3. Hart BL, Dudley MH, Zumwalt RE. Postmortem cranial MRI and autopsy correlation in suspected child abuse. *Am J Forensic Med Pathol*. 1996;17:217-224.

4. Feldman KW, Weinberger E, Milstein JM, Fligner CL. Cervical spine MRI in abused infants. *Child Abuse Negl*. 1997;21:199-205.

5. Thornton RN, Jolly RD. The objective interpretation of histopathological data: an application to the ageing of ovine bruises. *Forensic Sci Int.* 1986;31:225-239.

6. Raekallio J. Histological estimation of the age of injuries. In: Perper JA, Wecht CH, eds. *Microscopic Diagnosis in Forensic Pathology.* Springfield, Ill: Charles C Thomas; 1980:3-16.

7. Souviron R, Mittleman RE, Valor J. Obtaining the bitemark impression (mold) from skin: A technique for evidence preservation. *FBI Law Enforcement Bulletin.* 1982:8-11.

8. Gilliland MG, Folberg R. Shaken babies—some have no impact injuries. *J Forensic Sci.* 1996;41:114-116.

9. Hobbs CJ. Skull fracture and the diagnosis of abuse. *Arch Dis Child.* 1984;59:246-252.

10. Reece RM, See R. Childhood head injuries: accidental or inflicted? *Arch Pediatr Adolesc Med.* 2000;154:11-15.

11. Choux M, Grisoli F, Peragut JC. Extradural hematomas in children. 104 cases. *Childs Brain.* 1975;1:337-347.

12. Gennarelli TA, Meaney DF. Mechanisms of primary head injury. In: Wilkins RH, Rengachary SS, eds. *Neurosurgery.* New York, NY: McGraw-Hill; 1996:2611-2621.

13. Leestma JE. *Forensic Neuropathology.* New York, NY: Raven Press; 1988.

14. Duhaime AC, Gennarelli TA, Thibault LE, Bruce DA, Margulies SS, Wiser R. The shaken baby syndrome. A clinical, pathological, and biomechanical study. *J Neurosurg.* 1987;66:409-415.

15. Jenny C, Hymel KP, Ritzen A, Reinert SE, Hay TC. Analysis of missed cases of abusive head trauma [published erratum appears in *JAMA* 1999;282(1):29]. *JAMA.* 1999;281:621-626.

16. Case ME, Graham MA, Handy TC, Jentzen JA, Monteleone JA, for the National Association of Medical Examiners Ad Hoc Committee on Shaken Baby Syndrome. Position paper on fatal

abusive head injuries in infants and young children. *Am J Forensic Med Pathol.* 2001:22:112-122.

17. Adams JH, Doyle D, Ford I, Gennarelli TA, Graham DI, McLellan DR. Diffuse axonal injury in head injury: definition, diagnosis and grading. *Histopathology.* 1989;15:49-59.

18. Geddes JF, Whitwell HL, Graham DI. Traumatic axonal injury: practical issues for diagnosis in medicolegal cases. *Neuropathol Appl Neurobiol.* 2000;26:105-116.

19. McKenzie KJ, McLellan DR, Gentleman SM, Maxwell WL, Gennarelli TA, Graham DI. Is beta-APP a marker of axonal damage in short-surviving head injury? *Acta Neuropathol (Berl).* 1996; 92:608-613.

20. Gentleman SM, Roberts GW, Gennarelli TA, et al. Axonal injury: a universal consequence of fatal closed head injury? *Acta Neuropathol (Berl).* 1995;89:537-543.

21. Gleckman AM, Bell MD, Evans RJ, Smith TW. Diffuse axonal injury in infants with nonaccidental craniocerebral trauma: enhanced detection by beta-amyloid precursor protein immunohistochemical staining. *Arch Pathol Lab Med.* 1999;123:146-151.

22. Lindenberg R, Freytag E. Morphology of brain lesions from blunt trauma in early infancy. *Arch Pathol.* 1969;87:298-305.

23. Piatt JH Jr, Steinberg M. Isolated spinal cord injury as a presentation of child abuse. *Pediatrics.* 1995;96:780-782.

24. Gosnold JK, Sivaloganathan S. Spinal cord damage in a case of non-accidental injury in children. *Med Sci Law.* 1980;20:54-57.

25. Brown RL, Brunn MA, Garcia VF. Cervical spine injuries in children: a review of 103 patients treated consecutively at a level 1 pediatric trauma center. *J Pediatr Surg.* 2001;36:1107-1114.

26. Rooks VJ, Sisler C, Button B. Cervical spine injury in child abuse: report of two cases. *Pediatr Radiol.* 1998;28:193-195.

27. Thomas HN, Robinson L, Evans A, Bullock P. The floppy infant: a new manifestation of nonaccidental injury. *Pediatr Neurosurg.* 1995;23:188-191.

28. Geddes JF, Hackshaw AK, Vowles GH, Nickols CD, Whitwell HL. Neuropathology of inflicted head injury in children. I. Patterns of brain damage. *Brain.* 2001;124(pt 7):1290-1298.

29. McCormick WF. Pathology of closed head injury. In: Wilkins RH, Rengachary SS, eds. *Neurosurgery.* New York, NY: McGraw-Hill; 1996:2639-2666.

30. Willman KY, Bank DE, Senac M, Chadwick DL. Restricting the time of injury in fatal inflicted head injuries. *Child Abuse Negl.* 1997;21:929-940.

31. Levin AV. Retinal haemorrhages and child abuse. In: David TJ, ed. *Recent Advances in Paediatrics.* Vol 18. London, England: Churchill Livingstone; 2000:151-219.

32. Christian CW, Taylor AA, Hertle RW, Duhaime AC. Retinal hemorrhages caused by accidental household trauma. *J Pediatr.* 1999;135:125-127.

33. Betz P, Puschel K, Miltner E, Lignitz E, Eisenmenger W. Morphometrical analysis of retinal hemorrhages in the shaken baby syndrome. *Forensic Sci Int.* 1996;78:71-80.

34. Johnson DL, Braun D, Friendly D. Accidental head trauma and retinal hemorrhage. *Neurosurgery.* 1993;33:231-235.

FORENSIC INVESTIGATIONS

Det Bruce Foremny

— Suspect abuse any time children younger than age 4 years die from blunt force trauma not associated with motor vehicle collisions.

— Head trauma is the most common cause of death in blunt force trauma.

— Proof of child abuse must meet the same standards of evidence and testimony as used in the adult criminal justice system.

— Interagency or multidisciplinary protocols for investigators[1]:

1. Assist victims of child abuse through the judicial system with dignity and respect while minimizing secondary trauma.

2. Assist local law enforcement agencies with consistent investigation guidelines while recognizing local independence.

3. Mobilize the efforts of prosecutors, law enforcement, and medical, mental health, educational, and social service organizations to investigate, prevent, and address child abuse issues.

— To function on a multidisciplinary team, investigators must:

1. Understand their role.

2. Understand the family dynamics of domestic violence and child abuse.

3. Have a rudimentary knowledge of trauma medicine.

4. Understand the cause and effect of trauma on children.

5. Work with child protective services (CPS) to meet the child's immediate needs for protection, shelter, and emotional support.

6.   Understand the principles of prosecuting child abuse in the regional court system.

INITIAL RESPONSE TO HEAD TRAUMA

— Must report abusive or suspected head trauma to law enforcement and/or CPS organizations.

— Include provisions for protecting reporting sources against civil liability and allow for automatic cross-reporting between police and child welfare organizations.

— Perform scene assessments and interviews to support the pathologist's diagnosis of abusive head trauma (AHT) or sudden infant death syndrome.

— Most jurisdictions require investigations and autopsies for all unexpected child deaths.

FORENSIC PHOTOGRAPHY

— Be prepared to respond directly to the emergency department (ED) to take initial reports and obtain 35-mm and/or digital photographs of the victim's entire body.

1.   Show injuries, patterns or absence of injuries, and the child's overall condition.

2.   In fatal cases, take photographs to assist medical examiners in determining the cause, manner, and time of death.

3.   Take photographs at the time of the initial report and 24 and 72 hours after.

— Patterned injuries:

1.   Markings or bruises may take time to fully develop, so use a series of photographs to demonstrate development.

2.   Photographs help medical professionals explain injuries to juries and determine when and how injuries were inflicted.

— Use color film and include the entire child.

— Obtain detailed photographs of specific injuries with and without a color bar and scale, which allows accurate color film developing (in chemical photography) and scaled presentation of injuries.

— Do not ask physicians to date bruises based on color; bruises develop, discolor, and heal at varying rates.

— CPS requires that physicians conduct medical examinations of the siblings of child abuse victims.

1.   Assist by providing photographers during medical assessments.

2.   Photograph siblings in same manner as victims to help determine if the primary victim is the target child or one of several abuse victims.

— Instant cameras are not good substitutes for 35-mm color film or digital cameras.

— Take as many detailed, high-quality photographs as needed.

— Do not combine cases on the same roll of film or photo card to save money.

— Have film developed in police photography laboratories or contract photography laboratories with established reputations for preserving the dignity and integrity of police investigations.

— Maintain digital photographs on disks that are not rewriteable in order to safeguard against allegations of tampering.

DIGITAL PHOTOGRAPHY
— Images can be easily enhanced and manipulated by medical professionals to assess and discuss injuries in consultation with experts.

— Photographs can be used by prosecutors to decide whether to charge persons with abuse. Prosecutors can enhance, crop, or focus photographs for presentation at trial.

— For more information, see "Use of Digital Imaging and Photographs" in Chapter 12, Prosecution and Courtroom Issues.

HANDLING PHOTOGRAPHS
— It is improper and unprofessional to keep "trophy books" of police

investigations or to use victims' photographs for commercial or political exploitation.

— Images can help educate professionals involved in the investigation, treatment, prosecution, or prevention of child abuse; use judiciously.

INITIAL CASE ASSESSMENT REPORT

— Establish:

1. Level of suspicion for AHT.

2. Identity of suspected perpetrator and whether the perpetrator poses a risk for the victim.

3. Whether there are other children in the home.

4. Where the suspected abusive trauma occurred (jurisdiction).

5. How the medical staff believes the abusive trauma occurred.

6. When the medical staff thinks the abusive trauma occurred.

— ED nurses or social workers should obtain a complete history from the patient or caregivers.

1. The history is used to make medical assessments and treat injuries.

2. Review the medical history before interviewing caregivers or the family.

3. The history documents the interaction between the victim and caregivers.

4. Note who was providing care at the time of injury and the explanation given.

5. Note who the child is most and least comfortable with.

6. Note who had access to the child during the period beginning 72 hours before coming to the hospital until the symptoms of injury first appeared.

— Interview physicians for injury assessment to compare with family history.

1. Obtain the possible time frame for the injuries and narrow the time frame to weeks, days, or hours.

2. Determine the existence of other potential abusive injuries. Most hospital protocols require a suspected nonaccidental trauma radiographic series (skeletal survey).

— Rules of criminal procedure differ by state, but the diagnosis of battered child syndrome can be admissible at trial as a prior act indicating a pattern of behavior.

1. A prior act refutes defenses such as accidental injury or false identification of the offender.

2. It may also be useful if the defendant takes the stand.

3. Make information available to the prosecutor, who decides its potential value.

— Meet often with medical personnel to learn the language of the medical community.

1. A diagnosis is not static. It is a dynamic process based on changing findings.

2. Share information about the investigation as it becomes available so physicians can update findings.

3. Prosecutors or attorneys may ask that physician interviews be recorded to commit the physicians to a diagnosis. Rather than record these interviews, take detailed notes, review them at the end of the interviews, and provide rough drafts to the physicians for them to clarify and/or correct.

4. Often physicians add valuable points and enhance opinions with better medical language.

5. Recognize that medical opinions alone are insufficient to solve crimes or win convictions.

INITIAL INTERVIEW OF CAREGIVERS

— The purpose is to commit caregivers, families, and witnesses to a time frame for the injuries, indicating or eliminating potential witnesses and suspects.

— The interview may indicate where the injuries occurred and what instruments were used.

— The first contact with the child's family is crucial.

1. Show empathy, concern, and conviction that the truth is being sought.

2. Conduct interviews to gather facts to aid medical personnel and police in resolving the suspicion of abuse.

— Most initial interviews last 20 to 30 minutes and focus on reconstructing the last 72 hours of the child's life.

— Recorded initial interviews are not practical or proper, but some states allow taping without caregivers' knowledge or consent. This commits caregivers to their stories without placing unneeded stress on them or their families.

— Conduct initial interviews away from distractions.

INTERVIEW TECHNIQUES

— The best technique depends on the circumstances as well as the personality of the interviewer.

1. Find interview techniques that feel natural and comfortable.

2. If interview techniques are legal, moral, and ethical, use them.

3. Do not talk too much or listen too little.

— Coordinate efforts with CPS, especially noting prior contacts with the family.

— Conduct standard criminal histories and local records checks to uncover recent (within 1 calendar year) police contacts.

1. Record checks are done for officer safety as well as for insight into the family.

2. Reports of child abuse or neglect or incidents of domestic violence may reveal who acts violently in the home and under what circumstances.

3. Reports may also give an idea of the best approach for interviews.

— Police officers and detectives should identify themselves as such.

1. Most states allow latitude on how introductions are made.

2. Plainclothes detectives or investigators must be prepared to show photographic identification and should introduce themselves first as a person and then as an investigator.

3. Act with compassion toward caregivers and convey the role you play in the inquiry.

4. Help to put the family and caregivers at ease.

— Department policy and local custom dictate attire.

1. Many medical facilities prefer that weapons not be displayed.

2. Department policies and the situation dictate officer safety.

3. In initial interview settings, shed symbols of authority to avoid distracting the interviewee and reminding suspects that it is a police investigation with consequences for the guilty.

4. Be nonauthoritarian and unassuming.

5. The more comfortable caregivers, the family, and witnesses are, the more productive the initial interviews will be.

6. Use the victim's first name during interviews and listen to how caregivers, the family, and witnesses refer to the child.

— Interview caregivers, family members, or witnesses by themselves.

— If a second investigator is present, have that investigator remain in the background and act as an observer and note taker while you speak with the interviewee.

— Sit in a comfortable place close to the person being interviewed to establish an informal conversational setting.

— The second investigator should note body language and mannerisms.

— Obtain family history before discussing how injuries occurred.

1. Ask about chemical dependency, criminal history (both arrests and allegations), history of domestic violence or child abuse, family stresses such as finances or employment, and parentage of the victim.

2. Ask whether others in the home were abused.

3. Determine if the parents or babysitters are experienced and if the level of care needed by the victim is beyond their ability.

4. Ask questions that elicit narrative responses.

5. Avoid questions that require only a limited response or a "yes" or "no" reply.

6. Do not interrupt the narrative as long as the focus is on the issue at hand.

7. Keep the subject on the child.

8. Note if the interviewees are speaking tangentially to avoid answering questions or if it is simply in their nature.

— A semistructured cognitive interview technique employs open-ended, cue, and direct questions.

1. Elicit narratives by asking open-ended questions, then return to specific issues with cue questions to elicit further narrative about specific issues.

2. End with direct questions to elicit direct responses.

— Have a basic idea of the time frame for the injuries based on physicians' assessments.

1. In battered child syndrome, the child may have healed injuries or multiple injuries in various stages of healing.

2. Establish a time line and determine who had access to the victim during the injury time frame (72 hours before injury through coming to the hospital).

3. Carefully question caregivers about when the child became symptomatic.

— Ask caregivers about accidental traumas that went unreported.

— Provide information promptly to physicians to see if it changes the diagnosis or treatment.

DOCUMENTING THE CRIME SCENE

— Once a time line is established, locate the scene of the abuse.

1. Consider the scene the same as the scene of any other crime.

2. There may be multiple physical locations.

— Carefully assess the scene.

1. Use common sense plus training and experience.

2. Observe the scene and potential evidence from a long distance, an intermediate distance, and close up.

3. Those who are parents should rely on personal experiences to judge the feasibility of the history, but not the person who provided the history.

— Process the scene with photographs (**Figures 11-1-a** and **b; 11-2; 11-3; 11-4-a, b,** and **c;** and **11-5**). See also Chapter 12, Prosecution and Courtroom Issues.

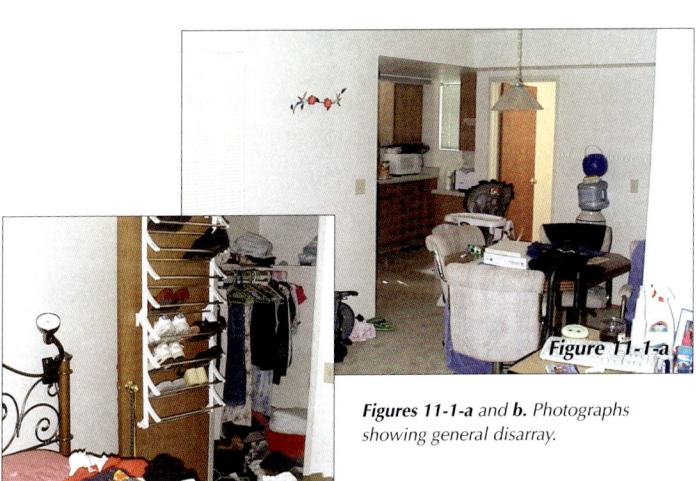

Figures 11-1-a and **b.** Photographs showing general disarray.

Figure 11-1-a

Figure 11-1-b

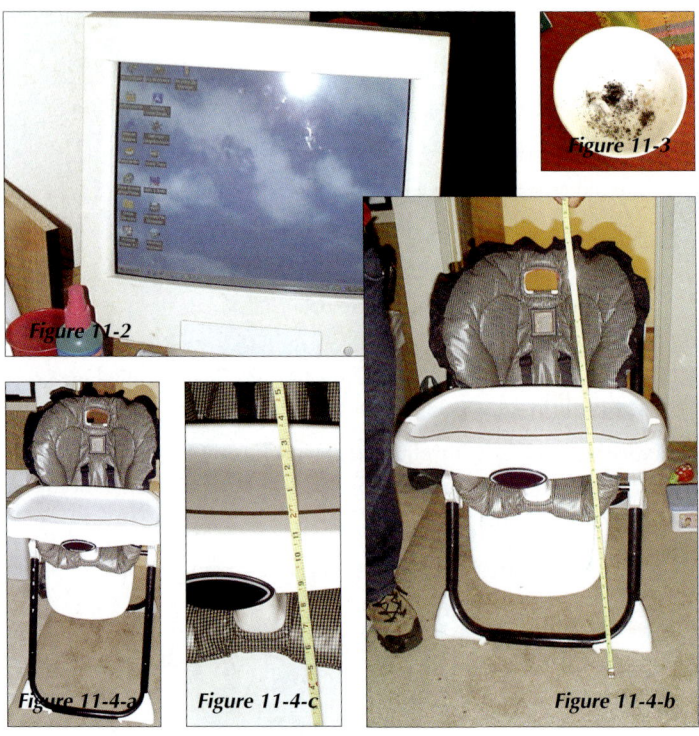

Figure 11-2. Computer as found by investigators. Photographs of a computer as found by the police can help refute allegations of police tampering. A trained forensic computer expert should be used to seize computers and computer files with a specially worded search warrant.

Figure 11-3. Evidence of tobacco use on front porch of an apartment that is supposed to be smoke-free and is occupied by a woman who claims to live alone and does not smoke.

Figures 11-4-a and *b.* A high chair at its maximum and minimum heights. Note the flooring in relation to the high chair and the separation between the linoleum tile in the kitchen and the carpeted dining area. By photographing both types of flooring, the investigator gives an accurate portrayal of the kitchen and dining areas, assisting the experts who may need to factor in the types of flooring when eliminating a parent's "accidental" explanation of a fall as the cause of a fatal injury.

Figure 11-4-c. The tape measure used by investigators is angled, giving an inaccurate measurement.

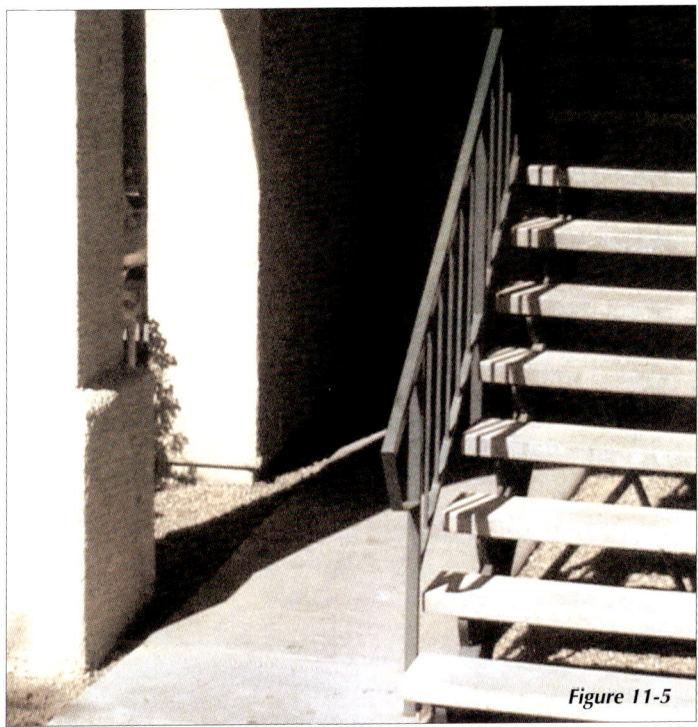

Figure 11-5. *View of front entrance to a crime scene (an apartment) from a witness's apartment. This perspective shows what the witness could have seen from his window at a distance of approximately 18m. In this photograph, the crime scene appears much closer than it actually is, due to the use of the zoom feature when it was taken, and the entrance to the crime scene is blocked by a shadow.*

— When abuse results in death, use photographs to document the presence of lividity, or pooling of blood in the body by way of gravity after death.

1. Lividity helps medical examiners determine the approximate time of death and whether the body was moved, altered, or staged.

2. A fixed *lividity* pattern can refute a perpetrator's story.

3. Consult medical examiners before confronting caregivers because lividity and rigor mortis develop in infants at a different rate than in adults.

— Attend the autopsy and assist medical examiners/coroners by providing data received while collecting and analyzing evidence.

— Be prepared to work along with medical examiners to find patterns or mechanism of injury.

— Patterned injuries are unlikely in blunt force head trauma.

— Nonsexual DNA and other trace evidence is of limited value.

— Look for foreign material.

— When it is suspected that the child's head or body was thrown into a hard surface, process that surface for hair, blood, tissue, or DNA.

— The most likely crime scene is the victim's or caregiver's home.

— Cases of child abuse usually involve no plan for concealment, excuse, or escape.

— Scene alteration may be prevented by committing suspects and witnesses to histories early and moving quickly to where the event occurred.

— Confront the caregiver to obtain either a confession or an altered history of the event.

— When the caregiver confesses to abuse, do not stop the investigation.

1. Take the confession in detail and compare it with the injuries.

2. Videotape the confession at the scene and have the suspect demonstrate the abuse.

   A. Allow medical experts to judge whether the confession is consistent with the injuries.

   B. The videotape is evidence for the court and can help dispel the belief that nice people never do such things to children.

PREMEDITATION

— Most child abuse is not planned, but premeditated abuse or murder does happen.

— Assume offenders have read materials related to AHT and its investigation.

— Look for evidence of where the crime was planned and where evidence is concealed.

— Offenders in child murders may stage crime scenes to look like abductions.

1. Consider gender.

   A. In the 1- through 5-year-old age group, male and female victims are equally at risk for family-related abduction.

   B. Boys aged 1 to 5 years are far more likely to be abducted by strangers than by family members; the opposite is true for girls in the same age group.

2. Consider who is reporting and the details of the abduction before ruling out in-home abuse.

HANDLING EVIDENCE

— If victims, witnesses, or suspects describe evidence, find and photograph it, then seize and preserve it for scientific examination or re-creation.

— If victims, witnesses, or suspects mention evidence that cannot be found, report it.

1. Look where suspects may have concealed items or attempted to have them destroyed (dumpsters, storage lockers, canals).

2. Even burned evidence may leave identifiable residue.

3. If items cannot be found, try to duplicate them and re-create conditions.

— Those grieving a child's death may act out violently against objects believed responsible.

— Child murderers may alter or destroy evidence.

— Act quickly to preserve evidence.

— If evidence is destroyed and suspects do not supply enough information for its replacement, look for receipts for or photographs of the item.

— While processing the scene, document and memorialize it in a narrative report accompanied by photographs.

1. Note the general condition of the residence, lighting, safety hazards, and temperature.

2. Rely on the report and not personal memory.

SEARCH WARRANTS

— The need for search warrants to process a crime scene varies by state.

— To determine if a search warrant is needed, ask the following questions:

1. Is this a crime?

2. Is there a known scene other than the victim's body?

3. Are there people who may be suspects and will they have expectations of privacy at the scene?

4. Do I have probable cause for a search warrant?

— Probable cause:

1. Is defined as facts and circumstances that would lead a reasonable person to believe that a crime has been committed and that evidence of that crime may be found at the place to be searched.

2. Prosecutors or state attorneys may authorize search warrants with investigators as affiants.

   A. Present the facts of the case in a simple, concise manner for prosecutors.

   B. Never embellish the facts or credentials to obtain a warrant. This can lead to negative legal consequences.

— Informed consent:

1. Law enforcement investigators should identify themselves as such.

2. Establish who has the domain and lawful authority to give consent to search specific areas or items in the home.

    A. A wife may give consent to search the home with the exception of areas that are the exclusive domain of the husband.

    B. A parent may give consent to search all common areas.

3. Ensure the consent is witnessed, recorded, or obtained in writing.

4. When a motion is filed to suppress evidence, the court usually requires the state to prove that the consent search was valid and the defense to prove that a search with a warrant was not valid. It is best to search a scene by warrant rather than consent.

— If a search warrant is obtained, still ask for consent to search.

1. If consent is refused, the search warrant still allows the search to take place, but the suspect may be forced to defend the refusal in court.

2. Having consent provides dual protection for evidence seized.

3. If the search warrant is judged flawed, consent ensures that the evidence is admissible.

— Consult with legal advisors or local prosecutors for more direction.

SEARCHING FOR WITNESSES

NEIGHBORHOOD CANVASS

— Canvassing involves conversations between investigators and the neighbors of the family in which the abuse occurred.

1. Canvasses can be conducted in any facility or neighborhood, regardless of income.

2. Neighbors hear and see things they may not tell police but may share if asked.

— Involve case agents in neighborhood canvasses.

1. May have to rely on personnel from other police units to assist in the search.

2. Consider training support teams on the mechanics of neighborhood searches.

— Searches are usually conducted in the early evening.

— If the media is following the case, conduct the search when they are not present.

— Prepare questions that elicit narrative responses.

— Caution personnel to listen carefully to responses.

— If relevant information is obtained, conduct a detailed interview and follow-up.

— Give neighbors flyers or business cards in case they remember something later.

1. Allows informants to remain anonymous

2. Provides a referral for potential witnesses who were not home at the time of the original search

— Silent witness programs:

1. Offer a reward for information leading to an arrest in a homicide case.

2. Advertise the reward during the search.

3. Provide a 24-hour phone number as well as the investigator's phone number.

4. Assign trained personnel to the 24-hour phone line to receive information during and immediately after the canvass.

— If the media complements the neighborhood canvass, keep phone lines staffed during newscasts.

— Examine information as it arrives or is uncovered, including data on callers and suspects.

— Involve beat officers or community action team members who know the neighborhood to advise and assist in the canvass.

1.   Include postal workers, maintenance workers, domestic staff, groundskeepers, or other people providing services to the family and interacting with them on a regular basis. They are often ignored as sources of information.

2.   Contact these people away from their place of employment.

3.   Involve schools, youth organizations, and churches.

    A. Siblings may attend local schools even if the victim is too young.

    B. Talk to teachers for insight into the family.

    C. Obtain similar data from the leaders of any organization to which the child belongs.

— Confidentiality mandates for churches and clergy vary between states and religions.

1.   Most allow clergy to report and discuss allegations of abuse involving a child as long as the information was not obtained during confession and does not violate the priest-petitioner relationship.

2.   Clergy members must assert confidentiality.

3.   Leaders of Bible study groups or Sunday school classes can have valuable information or disclosures from the family that do not violate the spirit of the confessional.

4.   Consult the local prosecutor for guidelines.

HISTORICAL DATA
— Obtain family history from family and neighbors.

1.   Prior allegations and investigations may show a cycle of violence and be used as prior acts. Admissibility varies from state to state.

2.   Information can be used in follow-up interviews and may prompt other charges.

3.   Present information to prosecutors so they can assess its value at trial.

— Obtain a complete criminal history to gain insight for future interviews.

1. Review police reports to assess the suspect's propensity to lie rather than confess when confronted with physical evidence or witness statements.

2. Intoxication is usually not a defense in violent crimes against children; offenders may try to blame chemical abuse for child abuse.

3. Not all who are abused as children grow up to be child abusers, but mentioning this tendency allows the offender to project blame while confessing to abuse.

— If the prior history involves the current family, this may provide insight into which family members lie or minimize the truth to protect the offender and which were intimidated to recant in court or refused to testify.

1. When prior abuse occurred with other family units, inform the current family of this history and possibly gain allies.

2. Use past behavior to predict future behavior.

    A. Without meaningful intervention, families experiencing domestic violence will continue the cycle of violence.

    B. The type of violence often remains the same.

3. Review mental health records.

— Prior investigation, arrest, or conviction in a criminal matter or civil dependency hearing may cause an offender to modify behavior to conceal abusive acts.

— Seek out records of CPS, local schools, churches, mental health facilities, hospitals, medical clinics, and calls for service within police agencies.

— If the family is reported for domestic violence or child abuse in a particular jurisdiction, they may move to others to avoid being prosecuted. Contact other jurisdictions and medical facilities for reports of domestic violence, child abuse, or suspected abusive trauma.

— Do not automatically discount unfounded or uncharged allegations of abuse from other jurisdictions or agencies.

— Be aware that CPS investigations may be closed because they could not establish the identity of the perpetrator.

1. Consider examining the medical evidence in prior allegations.

2. Inquire if a qualified pediatric radiologist evaluated the images. If not, consider having the evidence evaluated by a qualified professional.

3. Ascertain whether the police conducted proper follow-up interviews or if the case was closed when family members moved.

4. Some cases are closed when prosecuting authorities decline prosecution because of judicial economy.

— Determine if there is an established history of false reports made by a vindictive ex-spouse or if allegations were discounted.

1. Examine which came first, the divorce or the allegation of abuse, and if spousal abuse or child abuse could be the reason for the divorce.

2. Examine relationships with ex-spouses, ex-boyfriends, and ex-girlfriends and ascertain why they ended.

— Obtain prior medical records for the victim and other family members and look for a pattern of abuse and neglect. Any *exculpatory evidence* (evidence showing a suspect's innocence) must be given the same attention as *inculpatory evidence* (evidence showing a suspect's guilt).

— Pay attention to stories offered by caregivers to account for the injuries.

1. Sometimes a person offers the same story or a similar story in separate but similar instances.

2. Look for caregivers who modify their histories when speaking to sympathetic family members and friends.

3. Use inconsistent explanations in later confrontational interviews and present them in court as inconsistent statements if a caregiver takes the stand.

— The absence of a history of violent behavior does not preclude a potential suspect.

1. Many acts of abuse go unreported or undetected.

2. Some acts of abuse are committed by those who are too young to have a history with police, CPS, or social services.

INTERACTION WITH FIRST RESPONDERS

— Emergency medical services (EMS) reports are usually available to law enforcement personnel for child abuse investigations.

1. Written requests may be required by statute or grand jury subpoenas.

2. The reports provide valuable medical information from the first responders and usually contain the histories given by families or caregivers.

— Interview EMS and fire department personnel (**Table 11-1**).

1. EMS and fire personnel may need to alter a scene to preserve life.

2. Fire departments may be receptive to training on scene preservation in conjunction with treatment of victims.

Table 11-1. Questions That Should Be Asked of First Responders
1. What did you hear, see, touch, or smell at the scene?
2. What was the temperature of the room and the victim?
3. What did you do to the victim to assess, stabilize, and transport?
4. In a fatal situation, what did you move or alter on the body?
5. What was the condition of the house/apartment when you arrived?
6. What did the family/caregiver say or do while you were there?
7. Was there anything unusual?
8. Did the family do any clean-up or alterations that you saw?
9. Did you or your team move anything or do any clean-up?
10. What do you think happened here? Why?

3. Statements made to EMS personnel may be admissible under the hearsay exception if they were made spontaneously or elicited to further treatment.

4. Contact local state attorneys or prosecutors for guidance.

— EMS calls may be recorded on audiotape and kept for 30 days to 1 year.

1. Tapes can provide valuable evidence and are almost always admitted into court under the hearsay exception.

2. They can reveal the circumstances of the call for emergency medical assistance.

3. Callers are more likely to tell the truth or stage a quick lie to EMS personnel.

4. If possible, listen to the EMS tape before responding to the initial investigation or talk to EMS responders on their way to the hospital or scene.

5. Always listen to EMS tapes before interviewing suspects.

OBSERVATION AND CREATING A FOCUS

— Compile a list of people with access to the victim and note ability to inflict injuries.

1. Do not automatically eliminate people because of age, gender, profession, or religion.

2. May eliminate because of ability or disability.

3. Use knowledge, training, observation, and common sense to limit the suspect list to those who could reasonably be expected to have caused the injuries.

— Prioritize the list using family or caregiver histories and neighborhood searches, give medical professionals the information, and develop investigative focus.

1. Use common sense and observation to examine the most likely suspects.

2. Find witnesses.

3. Encourage the victim to disclose who committed the abuse.

4. Obtain a confession when possible.

— Do not depend on the medical community to solve the crime.

POLYGRAPH EXAMINATIONS

— Use reputable polygraph examiners who are experienced police investigators.

— Examiners should be members in good standing with the American Polygraph Association and/or the American Association of Police Polygraphists.

— Polygraphs eliminate those least likely to have inflicted injuries.

1. Fully brief examiners on the investigation and backgrounds of the suspects.

2. Most examiners conduct 2 polygraph examinations per day; consequently, the process will take several days if there are multiple suspects.

— Be available to examiners for a pretest interview to agree on questions to use.

1. A pretest interview may elicit statements from witnesses or suspects not previously known to investigators.

2. May eliminate the need for a polygraph examination or change the direction of the investigation.

— Remain available during the polygraph examination and after for posttest interviews.

1. This shows confidence in the process and enables the investigator to step into interviews to confront deceptive people.

2. Posttest interviews are the best times to obtain confessions.

3. Ensure the process is noncoercive.

— Polygraph examinations are not substitutes for good police work.

— Do not use routinely when investigations prove the witnesses' statements.

— Do not use for all suspects whose confession was validated.

— Overuse casts doubt on truthful statements already verified.

ELICITING STATEMENTS FROM SUSPECTS
See **Table 11-2**.

Table 11-2. Considerations in Head Trauma Abuse
— Victims from birth to the age of 5 years are most vulnerable and least likely to report. Most victims are younger than 1 year.
— The nature of the head injuries results in children being left brain-damaged or having fatal outcomes (25%), eliminating credible victim statements.
— Other children who witness the event may be nonverbal because of their age or may be difficult to interview.
— Witnesses to violent child abuse may be too afraid to talk, fearing that they might also be abused.
— Abuse is often not an isolated event and witnesses may have already been victims of abuse or domestic violence, making them afraid to cooperate with investigation.
— Some adult witnesses are so involved in the cycle of domestic violence that they may be afraid to disclose abuse or are themselves perpetrators of abuse. Adult witnesses who were not participants may fear consequences for not reporting earlier abuse.

PRETEXT OR CONFRONTATIONAL TELEPHONE CALLS
— These calls are used to obtain statements from the suspect early in the investigation.

— Enlist a civilian witness to call the suspect and solicit a confession.

— By manipulating the dialogue, the witness makes the suspect feel that, by winning the witness's trust, the witness can be manipulated and controlled to help conceal the crime or alter evidence.

— Obtaining a confession in this manner is legal if one person involved in the call knows the conversation is being recorded; check specific state law.

Guidelines
— During the call, the caller acts as an agent of the police, so no promises, threats, or coercion can be used.

— Use recorded phone lines to memorialize the call.

1. Use a good-quality recorder wired directly into the phone line.

2. Employ an electronics company that handles law enforcement needs to help set up proper equipment.

3. Wear headphones to listen to the call and direct the conversation.

— Select a participant already eliminated from the suspect list.

1. The participant must be mature and intelligent enough to act like a person who can be manipulated by the suspect but not be a threat.

2. Usually a female relative or mature child can perform very effectively.

3. The child must be old enough to read and mature enough to testify in court.

4. Male authority figures are generally not good subjects for confrontation calls because they are not perceived as easily manipulated.

— Phone numbers must not appear on caller ID displays as police department or government phone numbers.

1. If possible, the phone should be associated with a fictitious name, address, and phone number.

2. The phone should never be answered by police personnel who are not acquainted with confrontational calls.

— The call must take place where police intercoms, loudspeakers, radios, pagers, cell phones, or conversations are not distractions. Any quiet place where the phone call can be both recorded and monitored suffices.

— Use caution when suggesting confrontation calls to witnesses.

1. Uneducated witnesses might call friends or civil attorneys not familiar with local laws to ascertain if confrontation calls are legal. These phone calls could result in bad advice or warnings to suspects that calls may occur.

2. Some witnesses may call suspects to get their advice or warn them about the staged calls. These witnesses' vulnerability and mixed feelings about the suspects can be used when staging calls but can be devastating if suspects are warned.

3. Thoroughly explain that a confrontation call is a legal, moral, and ethical way to obtain the truth.

— Conduct the confrontation call when the suspect can be expected to be alone and vulnerable to manipulation. Late evening is the most common time.

— Meet with the witness for about 1 hour before the call.

— Create an outline for the witness to follow.

1. Have the witness write the outline so the handwriting is easy for the witness to read.

2. Use 2 colors, one for the witness and one for the investigator's notes.

3. Ask the witness to help create the outline and put the conversation into common speech.

   A. Use a greeting that clearly identifies the suspect.

   B. Carry on a general conversation that puts both witness and suspect at ease.

   C. Use key questions to elicit narrative responses, eliminate defense, and lead the suspect to explain the how, what, when, where, and why of the incident.

4. Train the witness to listen and let the suspect talk.

— If the suspect does not confess, direct the conversation to the suspect's explanation of the injuries.

1. It is likely that the suspect will tell stories that can be proved false.

2. Check stories against those given in previous interviews.

— Prepare the witness for challenges from the suspect.

1. It is usually legal for police and their agents to lie to suspects to further investigations.

2. Stress to witnesses that they are acting at police direction and are not liars, which is what the defense will charge.

3. Advise witnesses that when they are asked difficult questions, they should ask questions of their own.

— End the phone call with a closing that leaves the witness in a non-threatening, neutral position.

OTHER CONSIDERATIONS
— Conduct equipment checks immediately before a confrontation call.

1. Have the witness state information such as name, date, and time in a practice call, then play the tape to make sure it is working.

2. Record the call on the tape where the leader ends.

— Sit next to the witness during the conversation, write notes, and coach.

— Most audiotapes permit 30 to 45 minutes of conversation before they must be changed.

1. Use only 1 side of a tape to avoid confusion during duplication and transcription.

2. Coach the witness to cough or create a diversion so the change can occur without disrupting the conversation.

3. Anticipate tape changes.

— Discovery requirements vary by jurisdiction.

1. Tape recordings of confrontation calls must be maintained as original pieces of evidence even if no statements were obtained or the tape malfunctioned.

2. Copy the tapes for use in the investigation before logging them as evidence.

3. Ensure all conversations between the suspect and witness appear on tape.

4. The notes or outline used can be destroyed or maintained for case files, depending on jurisdictional mandates.

5. Most jurisdictions require pretrial disclosure of taped confrontation calls.

6. Use tapes to elicit confessions.

— Confrontation calls can provide enough description of injuries to allow physicians to form opinions on whether the injuries are consistent with statements.

— Public records laws vary by state.

1. Do not use taped confrontation calls to sensationalize cases or for political or personal gain.

2. Consult with prosecutors or state attorneys before making any taped statements available to the media.

— The concept of a confrontation call can be applied to meetings between the suspect and civilian witness, but the risk to the witness is great.

1. Provide adequate police protection during in-person interviews.

2. Use sophisticated recording equipment with wireless receivers.

CONFESSIONS

— The purpose of suspect interrogations is to elicit truthful and verifiable confessions or equally damaging and verifiable lies.

— A confession can be obtained out of custody, in custody, or by telephone.

— Miranda warning or advice of constitutional rights:

1. Must always be given if the suspect is in custody and not free to leave.

2. Timing varies by jurisdiction.

3. If in doubt about whether Miranda rights apply, consult with local prosecutors or state attorneys before interviews.

4. If these resources are not available, advise suspects of their constitutional rights.

5. Give warnings verbally or in written form.

6. Ensure that you can prove that suspects understand their rights.

    A. Ask follow-up questions to elicit narrative responses.

    B. Include the responses in the report.

— During a confession, the suspect may give a heartfelt admission and show regret.

1. Suspect may confess when confronted by facts if shown compassion and understanding.

    A. Confessions are simple, direct, and easy to verify when compared to the medical evidence.

    B. An individual may demonstrate the abuse but minimize the force used.

2. A confession may also be obtained after several denials or false accounts.

    A. Feign belief in the lies and then confront the suspect, causing a change in the story until the truth is told.

    B. Even if the suspect never confesses, inconsistent statements and lies may be used at trial and can be hard to defend before a jury.

— Most jurisdictions uphold the use of trickery or deceit and do not invalidate confessions obtained in this manner.

— Do not be deterred or prejudiced by citizens who request attorneys or refuse to answer questions.

1. To overcome fears, become known in the community as honest and hardworking.

2. Do not end an investigation when suspects, family members, or caregivers invoke their constitutional right to remain silent or be questioned only with an attorney present. Suspects may still lie.

— Regarding keeping cases open or solving them without confessions:

1. Be patient with persons who invoke their rights. Nothing is lost by allowing attorneys to be present during questioning.

2. Prosecutors may recommend that investigators include them in contacting suspects' attorneys to arrange for interviews.

3. Attorneys representing witnesses often allow these interviews to occur and may even assist in obtaining information.

4. Interviews with attorneys present are better than no interview at all.

5. Whether invocations come from suspects, family members, or caregivers, maintain the possibility of future interviews by leaving business cards and asking them to call if they change their mind.

— Disclosure of recording equipment to suspects or witnesses varies with jurisdiction.

1. Contact the department's legal advisor, local prosecutor, or state attorney for guidance.

2. It is highly recommended that equipment be concealed so investigators can carry on general conversations or rapport building.

3. If the suspect refuses to be recorded but agrees to the interview, conduct the interview.

4. Involve a second investigator to take notes and act as a witness to statements.

5. Review the suspect's statements to allow the suspect to correct or clarify.

— If the suspect offers a confession or an explanation of the injuries, ask the suspect to make a written statement. Avoid dictating the statement or confession, but use notes from the interviews to refresh the suspect's recollection.

1. May take the form of a letter to the judge or victim explaining what happened and why or an apology to the victim or family.

2. Tell the suspect that the letter can and will be read by the judge, jury, defense counsel, prosecutor, and victim.

— If the suspect continues to offer lies in a confirmed case of AHT, listen to the suspect's statement and do not confront the lies.

1. Share medical opinions or other statements and evidence that discount the lie.

2. Remind the suspect that the lies will be proved wrong in court.

3. Conceal emotion and accept the suspect's attempts to minimize and rationalize behavior.

— Video equipment:

1. Ensure the suspect's demonstration of the cause of injury is visible to the camera.

2. Use dolls or other types of props.

3. Permit medical experts to use videotapes and give their opinions of whether the confession/history is consistent with the injuries.

THE MEDIA AND INVESTIGATIONS

— Be prepared for media attention.

— Follow agency policies governing statements made during ongoing investigations.

— Employ public information officers (if available) to handle the media or information requests.

— Coordinate with local prosecutors or state attorneys and, if possible, public information representatives.

— Keep the community focused on the injuries to or death of the child instead of allegations that can benefit the suspect.

— Educate superiors on the importance of completing the investigation before alerting the media.

PRESENTING CASES TO PROSECUTORS OR STATE ATTORNEYS

— See also Chapter 12, Prosecution and Courtroom Issues.

— Present all investigations of unexplained or abusive trauma to local prosecutors or state attorneys, who decide if criminal charges are warranted.

— Organize an investigation logically, usually chronologically.

— Separate medical records, CPS reports, photographs, transcripts, and recordings into binders for easy access and review.

— Present the case personally to offer oral overviews.

— If circumstances and the quality of the investigation meet the prosecutor's filing standards, the matter may be presented to a grand jury and/or at a preliminary hearing (see Chapter 12, Prosecution and Courtroom Issues).

— If called to testify to a grand jury or at a preliminary hearing, review the case carefully.

— The state attorney or prosecutor will decline to prosecute if the investigation is complete but no state laws have been violated.

— State attorneys or prosecutors who determine the need for further investigation should submit a request in writing.

1. Postfiling requests may be made with phone calls directing simple follow-up before probable cause hearings.

2. Keep commitments to complete such postfiling investigations.

— Police must consult the prosecutor before an arrest is made in some jurisdictions.

— In others, the prosecutor has 48 hours after an arrest to file charges before the suspect is released.

— In all jurisdictions, the filing decision is made when the investigation is complete.

PRETRIAL DISCOVERY AND PREPARING FOR TRIAL

— Know pretrial discovery requirements for your jurisdiction. Be prepared to conform to the jurisdiction's requirements where the case will be prosecuted.

— If pretrial interviews are required, prepare for them as if testifying in court.

1. Consider having prosecutors present.

2. Defense attorneys may wish to record interviews.

3. If allowed, also record the interviews for investigative benefit.

— Any pretrial statements made by investigators can be used as impeachment material at trial.

— State on tape that if the defense intends to use transcripts of interviews at court proceedings, copies should be available to review for accuracy at least 3 days before court proceedings.

— In pretrial interviews, be cooperative, concise, and accurate.

1. The content of pretrial interviews can cause the defense to seek out-of-court settlements (plea agreements).

2. Information intended to prove the suspect's guilt should be made available at pretrial interviews or it could be suppressed at trial.

3. See Chapter 12, Prosecution and Courtroom Issues.

ASSISTING PROSECUTORS AT TRIAL

— An investigator's job is not complete when the case is filed or an arrest is made.

— The defense may allege new facts that require verification.

— Be prepared:

1. To assist in locating and transporting witnesses.

2. To help prosecutors understand the facts of the case.

3. To provide a time line for the acts or counts of the indictment.

4. To prepare photographs, evidence, diagrams, or other exhibits for presentation to the judge and jury.

— Courts recognize case agents and allow exceptions to the exclusionary rule, making it possible for case agents to sit with prosecutors at trial.

— Maintain a neutral and professional demeanor regardless of what witnesses or the defense may say.

1. Do not respond to attacks by defense attorneys with negative body language, facial expressions, or verbal statements; jurors are watching.

2. Prosecutors will allow you to defend the process during your testimony.

— Maintain good posture as you approach the clerk to be sworn in, and while being sworn in stand straight and make eye contact with the clerk.

— Jurors must view investigators as serious professionals who have important things to say but who are fair and interested in finding the truth.

— Make eye contact with jurors, listen to questions to ensure you understand, and pause before answering to consider the answer and to allow for objections from the other side.

— Turn to jurors to answer questions.

1. Simple eye contact with jurors adds credibility.

2. Answer in complete sentences while looking from juror to juror.

— Teach the police or others in order to become comfortable speaking to juries about the subject matter. Opportunities for public speaking will raise comfort levels for persons in this role.

— Investigations can take place over months or years.

1. It is possible to be involved in as many as 50 different investigations in a year.

2. Use case reports to refresh your recollection.

3. Organize case files for trial to differentiate witnesses, suspects, and personal activities.

4. Read investigations and be familiar with all the information used.

5. If mistakes are made, correct them immediately or bring them to the attention of prosecutors so they can be corrected.

6. Maintain a resume detailing education, training, experience, and how many cases of suspected abusive injury you have worked.

    A. When considering the number cases worked, do not limit the number to only child abuse cases.

    B. Never embellish your credentials.

— After a conviction, you may still be called to assist the prosecution.

1. Sentencing recommendations

2. Mitigation and aggravation hearings

    A. Are similar to jury trials. Experts, family members, and members of the community may speak, asking for more or less severe sentences for defendants.

    B. Remain unbiased.

ASSISTING CHILD FATALITY REVIEW TEAMS

— Teams are established at both state and county levels.

— Comprise physicians, medical examiners, child development specialists, police investigators, and prosecutors.

— Collect timely and accurate data for the prevention, investigation, and prosecution of fatal injuries to children.

— Responsible for child helmet, pool fencing, and gunlock laws as well as recommendations on building better cribs, car seats, etc.

— Provide training in the investigative process for trauma doctors, local coroners, and CPS workers.

— Release criminal investigations, medical records, and coroners' reports to review teams.

COLD CASE INVESTIGATIONS

— Must examine old case files and photographs, medical examiner reports, original CPS investigations, and follow-up by social services.

— Sometimes a check of criminal histories or vital statistics reveals other abuse investigations or unexplained child fatalities.

— Examine histories of families, caregivers, and suspects.

— Have information reviewed by medical experts and pathologists who can apply contemporary knowledge to give direction or more conclusive diagnoses for injuries and time frames for traumatic events.

— Ascertain the availability of witnesses, family members, and the original suspects once a case is reopened.

— Recognize that completed investigations can bring closure to families or prove the innocence of suspects.

— Consider confrontation calls between suspects and nonthreatening family members, old friends, or anyone else willing to assist.

— Interview anyone who knew suspects before, during, or after abuse.

— Track any and all acts of violence committed by suspects before, during, and after fatal events.

— Interview suspects and confront them with all details of investigations.

— Present these cases in a manner similar to fresh ones.

1. Be prepared to testify in court about the evolution of police practices that led to the delayed completion of the investigation so jurors understand the difference between new information and faulty police work.

2. Notify families of victims as soon as possible, allowing them time to process outcomes before they are made public.

REFERENCE

1. Romley RM, for the Interagency Council, Maricopa County Children's Justice Project. *Multidisciplinary Protocol for the Investigation of Child Abuse*. Maricopa, Ariz: Interagency Council; 2004.

Chapter 12

PROSECUTION AND COURTROOM ISSUES

James R. Lauridson, MD
Robert N. Parrish, JD

— Cases of abusive head trauma (AHT) involving young victims often must be proved beyond any doubt because jurors and judges cannot believe that any "normal" person could engage in such violence and will often accept even implausible alternative explanations.

— Prosecutors must educate triers of fact and emphasize critical medical evidence using experts, visual demonstrations, and illustrative aids.

TEAM APPROACH

— Experienced child abuse prosecutors recommend working with investigators from the initial report of abuse until the trial and sentencing process are concluded.

— The same prosecutor should remain throughout all stages.[1]

— Prosecutors need basic education on the medical issues found in abuse, specifically, which injuries are consistent with accidental versus abusive trauma.

EXPERT CONSULTANTS

— Identify expert consultants early in the case.

— Consultants may suggest diagnostic tests to support an accurate opinion of what happened.

— Request a case conference with all medical experts and consultants to reach a consensus on the cause, mechanism, and timing of the injuries.

— Speak with peers or contact the American Prosecutors Research Institute's National Center for Prosecution of Child Abuse for referral to experts (http://www.ndaa.org/apri or 703-732-0321).

CHARGES AND CRIMES

— Decide whether the evidence identifies who committed the abuse and what that person's mental status was at the time.

1. Include elements related to the act performed (*actus reus*) and the intent to commit it (*mens rea*).

2. There is no crime committed if either element remains unproved beyond a reasonable doubt when the prosecution completes the presentation of evidence.

— Defense attorneys seek to establish reasonable doubt about defendants' guilt.

1. Consider the weight of evidence from different perspectives and decide what mental state fits the nature of the conduct.

2. Consider medical findings, statements made by suspect(s), and other direct or circumstantial evidence.

— Determine whether evidence indicates repeated abuse over time or a single incident.

— Decide whether to charge a separate count for each injury inflicted.

1. If the evidence shows the perpetrator had an isolated loss of impulse control, charge a lesser crime than if the injuries were inflicted in an extended beating.

2. Some states are debating whether causing permanent loss of brain function should be considered the same level of crime as causing death.

3. Consider the violence of the assault, even with good recovery. Many long-term consequences only become clear when the child begins schooling or organized athletics.

4. Consider the disparity in size and strength between the perpetrator and victim.

5.   Choose between charging the perpetrator for assault or waiting to determine the victim's ultimate outcome.

6.   Address the issue of the statute of limitations.

7.   Prosecutors must determine charges after considering all competing interests and explain the constitutional requirements for their choices.

DETERMINING WHO COMMITTED THE CRIME

— Various factors lead to identifying perpetrators (**Table 12-1**).

— Repeated abuse narrows the field of possible suspects to family members and regular childcare providers or babysitters.

Table 12-1. Factors to Consider in Determining Who Committed the Crime

—   Whose stories accounting for the injuries do not fit the severity of the child's injuries?

—   Which caregiver was with the child when symptoms first appeared?

—   Whose story changed to fit new information?

—   Who delayed in seeking medical care?

—   Which caregiver had a motive to hurt or kill the victim?

—   Who has unrealistic, age-inappropriate expectations of the child or other children?

—   Which caregiver was overstressed?

—   Who has a history of abusing this child or other children, of domestic violence, or of abusing animals?

—   Which caregiver must be in control?

—   Who blames other young children for inflicting the injuries?

—   Who caused caregivers to seek medical care from multiple and disparate providers?

—   Was one of the caregivers an abuse victim?

(continued)

> **Table 12-1.** *(continued)*
>
> — Was one caregiver critical of another caregiver's leniency with the child?
>
> — Has one caregiver provided a "partial admission"?
>
> — Who has shown little emotion about the injured child?
>
> — Who was alone with the child when suspicious or ill-explained injuries occurred?
>
> — Who calls the child "it," "him," or "my baby," but does not use the child's name?
>
> — Which caregiver is physically capable of inflicting the injuries?
>
> — Which caregiver is constantly seeking attention?
>
> — Has one caregiver blamed the young child or infant victim for the injuries?

1. It is challenging to determine the perpetrator in cases involving less severe head injuries.

2. In some cases involving repeated injury, the theory of accomplice liability may allow charging more than 1 caregiver, often with the same crime as the primary abuser.

CHARGING NONABUSIVE PARTNERS

— Criminal statutes may allow charges against caregivers who know about abuse and permit it to continue even though they probably did not cause injury.

— Determine whether nonabusers are capable of protecting themselves or the children in the context of the abuser's violence.

— Battered woman syndrome is not admissible as a defense in child abuse.[2]

— Factors in charging the nonabuser:

1. Type of abusive injuries

2. Whether the caregiver would have seen the injuries during daily caregiving

3.   Whether explanations offered by the abuser are obviously false

— Assess each case in light of its unique facts.

DECIDING TO PLEA BARGAIN

— Prosecutors may allow perpetrators to enter a guilty plea while still maintaining factual innocence.

— *Alford plea.* Defendant does not admit committing the crime but enters a guilty plea to avoid the consequences of being convicted at trial.

— *No contest plea.* Defendant does not admit committing the crime but acknowledges that the government has enough evidence to secure a conviction.

1.   These pleas are useless to the general aims of the criminal justice system in AHT cases.

2.   Lack of admission almost guarantees that any behavioral treatment will be ineffective.

— It is best to obtain some admission by the perpetrator, even if the plea entered is to a lesser offense.

MEETING WITH EXPERTS TO ADVANCE MEDICAL KNOWLEDGE

— It is often required in plea bargains that perpetrators meet with physicians, describe and demonstrate what they did to cause the injuries, discuss the triggering factors, and explain what happened after the child was injured.

1.   Videotape descriptions and demonstrations for later educational use.

2.   Videotaping guarantees that the defendant's admission is genuine and fits what is known by medical science before the judge accepts a plea of guilt.

3.   It is an incentive to give an honest account of the abusive conduct. If experts reject the explanation, the plea bargain fails.

4.   A polygraph test may further verify the accuracy of the account (see Chapter 11, Forensic Investigations).

BALANCING THE NEEDS OF THE PUBLIC, VICTIMS, AND DEFENDANTS

— The criminal justice system seeks a just result for victims by identifying and punishing perpetrators.

— Victims/families also have needs, goals, and a right to expect adequate and swift punishment of the perpetrator.

— Addressing the needs of criminal defendants:

1. The prosecution should resist the defense attorney's efforts to focus all attention on such needs at sentence hearings.

2. Consider the circumstances of the crime, the background and future of the defendant, and the overall interests of justice.

PRIMARY EXPERTS FOR THE PROSECUTION

— Criminal cases:

1. Jurors usually have little or no prior knowledge of medical or scientific issues and prosecutors have little time to educate them.

2. Select expert witnesses to educate jurors and prepare these experts to testify.

— Use visual depictions of concepts and physiologic processes.

— Decide which expert medical witnesses are needed to convey essential findings without unduly confusing or replicating testimony.

1. Most rules of evidence allow 1 or 2 experts to convey findings.[3,4]

2. Calling more experts increases the chance of introducing inconsistencies.

— In fatal cases, expert opinions from at least 1 pathologist and 1 clinician are necessary.

EXPERT EDUCATION OF THE TRIER OF FACT

GENERAL EDUCATION FOR THE JURY OR JUDGE

— Establish the qualifications of the expert witness.

— Explore battered child syndrome; shaken baby syndrome, or other forms of AHT; the diagnostic process for finding the cause and timing of injuries; medical research on the effects of common falls and other accidental trauma; the timing and onset of symptoms after certain injuries; and, when appropriate, information on perpetrators and common behaviors of child abusers.

— Detail the basic anatomy, structure, and function of infant/toddler brains; anatomy, structure, and function of the eyes; and mechanisms of head and eye injuries.

— The general education of the jury will differ depending on the combination of injuries.

— Include information on the effects of trauma on the brain, what symptoms would appear following infliction of the trauma, and how soon those symptoms would manifest.

— Offer appropriate visual depictions of medical concepts and issues.

— Jurors who see clear and credible graphics are less likely to be swayed by contradictory testimony, especially with no equally persuasive graphic presentations to support such testimony.

USE OF DIGITAL IMAGING AND PHOTOGRAPHS

Digital Imaging Basics

— Digital images are composed of pixels.

1. The term *pixel dimensions* refers to the number of vertical and horizontal pixels in an image.

2. Resolution improves with more pixels. An image with low resolution has a small number of pixels.

— Digital images are stored as computer files.

1. The size of the file increases as the number of pixels and amount of color information in each pixel increases.

2. The size of a color file depends on the amount of color information for each pixel (bit depth). With higher bit depth, more colors are displayed.

— Compression:

1. The computer scans the image for areas that are the same and

compresses them. When viewed, the computer automatically decompresses the file and displays the image.

2. Types of file compression:

   A. *Lossless compression.* The original file may be recovered in its original form. A common form of lossless compression is the *TIFF format* with LZW compression.

   B. *Lossy compression.* The compression process causes loss of image quality and detail not always recoverable. The most common form is the *JPG format.*

3. Visible image degradation occurs when a file is compressed repeatedly using the JPG format.

4. Even with degradation, if an expert witness verifies the image is accurate, it is admissible as evidence.

— Preserve the original image; any processing should be performed only on a copy.

1. Brightness/contrast, hue, and sharpening changes influence original data.

2. The quality of data and scientific knowledge at the foundation of computer graphics and animation of medical topics affects the graphics' quality.

3. Internal injuries require depiction of the relevant body part, location of injury, and potential mechanisms of injury.

4. Use an artist with medical training and experience to maximize accuracy in computer graphics.

— Judges should exclude misleading, speculative, or unsupported graphics.

— The ultimate test of computer graphics is whether the expert witness can lay the appropriate legal foundation for the graphics.

Teaching Graphics
— Present general concepts without dealing with case specifics.

— Can range from simple diagrams and animations to illustrate basic human anatomy to more complex diagrams and animations to teach more complex medical concepts.

— Must be accurate and consistent with current research and widely accepted scientific findings.

— Use to explain equations and physical principles.

— Rules for use of computer graphic demonstrations:

1. If graphics are intended to solely illustrate and clarify the testimony of an expert witness, they are admitted in the same way as any other chart, diagram, or drawing.

2. Graphics used to educate triers of fact need only reflect experts' opinions and be scientifically supported.

— Most courts in the United States recognize the legal status of computer animations as the same as experts' drawings on chalkboards or flip charts.

Case-Specific Graphics

— Present the evidence or injury patterns specific to the case being tried (**Figures 12-1** to **12-3**).

— Case-specific graphics are particularly useful with multiple injuries or complex evidence.

— The legal foundation for use is that they accurately depict the original injuries, as documented on radiographs, at autopsy, or on hospital photographs, and allow experts to better explain and illustrate opinions regarding the nature, location, timing, and cause of injuries.

— These graphics are treated the same as any other photograph, radiograph, or drawing.

— It is usually not required to establish how graphics were created as long as a comparison with underlying evidence shows they reasonably depict original findings.

— If it is claimed that the computer animation reenacts exactly what happened, the scientific reliability of the demonstration, the facts on

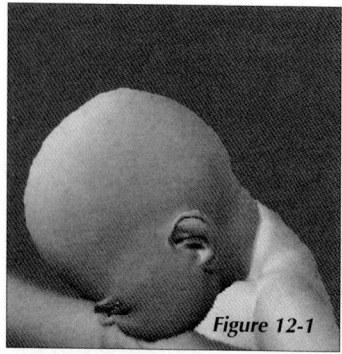

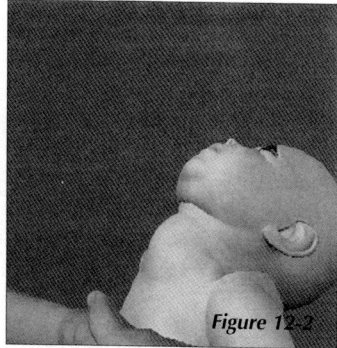

Figures 12-1 *and* **12-2.** *Illustrations of the movement of the infant's head and placement of the adult's hands during shaking.*

Figure 12-3. *Illustration of subdural hematoma and bridging veins.*

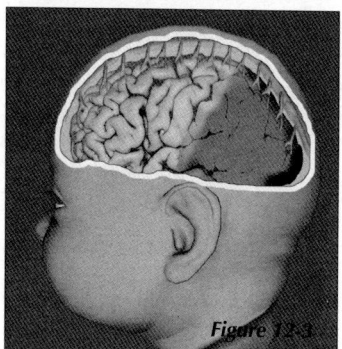

which it is based, and the opinion of the expert witness must be shown specifically.

1. The final arbiters are the expert witnesses.

2. Experts must testify that the animation accurately depicts the state of knowledge in the medical field regarding the type of forces needed to cause the particular injury.

3. Experts should acknowledge that the animated theory is not the only possible scenario.

4. Trial judges decide whether animated graphics can be shown to the jury.[5]

— Case law restricts the use of autopsy photographs showing the brain, subdural bleeding, ocular injuries, or abdominal injuries.

1.   These photographs must have "unusual probative value" to overcome the presumption of unfair prejudicial value.[6]

2.   Show original photographs to judges in pretrial motions to determine the accuracy and admissibility of computer graphics.

Simulation Graphics

— Simulations attempt to show exactly what happened in a given case, applying strict scientific principles to generate computer images.

1.   Will undergo close court scrutiny if challenged by the opposing party

2.   Must have a solid foundation in accurate, detailed measurements and, when appropriate, the concurrence of an accident reconstructionist, biomechanical engineer, or physicist

— AHT cases often have too many variables for a computer simulation program to accurately analyze all facts and generate an exact re-creation.

— Animation may be admissible if experts establish the proper foundation and can offer adequate explanations.

Mechanics of Presentation Graphics

— Basic hardware for graphic presentations should include a laptop computer and a projector able to project computer output.

1.   Desirable features of a presentation projector include portability, a bright display (light output greater than 1000 lumens), a large dynamic range of light output, keystone correction, manual focus, and manual zoom.

2.   XGA projectors have excellent resolution.

3.   Need a moderate-speed CPU, moderate RAM memory, a moderately-sized hard drive, CD-ROM drive, and high-resolution graphics.

4.   Test components together before purchasing.

— A commonly used presentation program is Microsoft PowerPoint.

More sophisticated graphics must be developed in specialized graphics packages and then incorporated into PowerPoint.

— Create and circulate a written operating procedure for storing images.

1. Valid operating procedure includes immediate transfer of original images to an unalterable medium, usually a CD-R (write-only) disc.

2. Before an image is written permanently to CD-R, rename it using a name with archival meaning.

ESTABLISHING THE MECHANISM AND TIMING OF INJURIES
— Victim's specific injuries:

1. The general education provided should dovetail with the actual injuries discussed by the experts.

2. Illustrate injuries in a way that jurors can understand and relate back to their general education.

— Presentation of injuries:

1. Organize injury presentation by body part. First discuss injuries to the head and eyes; second, the extremities (arms and legs); and third, the upper and lower torso.

2. Individually label/number structures for consistent use during trial.

— Ask expert witnesses about the significance of the injuries and likely mechanisms that could cause them.

— Guide experts to express opinions concerning the timing and onset of symptoms.

1. Question experts about the significance of an injury in conjunction with all the other injuries to the child.

2. Be aware that defense attorneys isolate each injury and have experts list all possible causes. Focus attention on the entire constellation.[7]

— Ask experts about the mechanism and degree of violence needed to cause the injuries.

1. It is rare to be able to specify a single possible mechanism.

2. Ocular damage, subdural or subarachnoid bleeding over the brain, axonal damage, and severe brain swelling occur in specific patterns only with severe, violent shaking.

3. Illustrate differences for juries so they can discern whether injuries occurred accidentally or intentionally.

— Expert medical opinions concerning timing are only complete and accurate if all facts are considered.

1. Blood on computed tomography scans of the brain are generally characterized as acute (less than 3 days old), subacute (up to 7 days old), or chronic (more than 7 days old).

2. Fractures are notoriously difficult to date.

— With more serious injuries, it is easier to prove who committed the abuse.

— With less serious injuries, symptom onset could take some time or be more subtle.

ESTABLISHING WHO COMMITTED THE ABUSE

— Ask expert medical witnesses questions to narrow the time frame of the injuries and establish the degree of violence involved.

1. Ask hypothetical questions concerning the victim's behavior before and after the injury, providing evidence of possible symptoms.

2. Ask experts when the injury was likely caused.

— When experts are allowed to testify about battered child syndrome, they may be qualified to offer direct opinions about the perpetrator.

— There are 2 common aspects of abuser behavior in battered child syndrome.

1. Perpetrators often delay seeking medical treatment for the victims.

2. It is common for the abuser to offer false stories to account for the injuries.[8]

ANTICIPATING AND RULING OUT ALTERNATIVE THEORIES
— Primary experts anticipate and explain why alternative theories of causation, mechanism, or timing of injuries are implausible or highly unlikely.

1. During the pretrial discovery phase, obtain court orders that the defense disclose the identity and substance of testimony of all proposed expert medical witnesses, including reports expressing experts' opinions.

2. Ask experts to explain why the injuries are not consistent with the defendant's story.

3. Ask experts to comment on theories proposed by the defendant's experts.

— Defense strategies:

1. The defense will ask the prosecution's medical experts if they can "exclude the possibility that . . ." or can say with 100% certainty that nothing other than shaking or shaking with impact could have caused the injuries.

2. Often experts acknowledge that alternative causes are at least possible.

3. Plausible explanations may raise reasonable doubt.

— Avoid being too closely tied to a particular medical theory as an explanation of injuries.

1. The primary burden for the prosecution is to prove a crime was committed by someone and prove beyond a reasonable doubt that the defendant is that person.

2. The exact mechanism of injury is rarely an element of the crime.

MEDICAL AND NONMEDICAL ASPECTS OF THE DEFENDANT'S CASE
ALIBI, CHARACTER, AND OTHER DEFENSE WITNESSES
— Defendants often call character witnesses to explain that they are

peaceful people, loving, wonderful parents, and not the type to harm children.

1. Prosecutors argue that such character witnesses' opinions are irrelevant.

2. Trial court judges usually permit this testimony and the rules of evidence generally support its introduction.[9]

3. Prosecutor's perspective:

    A. Ask witnesses if they have been with the defendant 24 hours a day, 7 days a week.

    B. Ask witnesses for their perceptions of people who could abuse children.

— Defense witnesses may claim defendants were not alone with the child long enough to have caused serious or fatal head injuries; however, it does not take long to cause such injuries.

— Defense witnesses who were with the defendant shortly before or after the injuries were allegedly inflicted may state that the defendant was acting normally and did not seem upset or stressed. In reality, there is no particular expected behavior of perpetrators before or after assaults. It is impossible to make any prediction based solely on behavior.

— Extended family members may testify that the defendant is a perfect parent.

1. Often a family history of stress is admitted because family members do not see it as connected to the abuse.

2. Family members can talk about the disciplinary methods used in the defendant's family.

— Defense witnesses may testify that the victim was particularly easy to care for and could not have triggered an assault; however, the act of abusing a child may be unrelated to the child's behavior.

NOTE: This testimony may contradict the experience and common sense of jurors.

CROSS-EXAMINATION OF DEFENDANTS

— Defendants typically testify in serious child physical abuse or homicide cases.

— They usually believe jurors will trust their account of the event, see how little they fit a criminal profile, and therefore decide against conviction.

— Attacking the defendant is not a wise strategy.

— Address inconsistent statements.

— Try to obtain admissions that the defendant was the primary caregiver for the child during the time of injury and that the defendant may have been under stress when the injuries were inflicted.

— Defendants may demonstrate in court what they saw or assume happened.

1. May show how alleged "shaking" to revive the child was accomplished.

2. Question defendants about why the child was unresponsive in the first place.

MEDICAL WITNESSES FOR THE DEFENSE

— Medical witnesses are called to offer scientific support of alternative causes for injuries.

— The defense may call medical experts to insist severe impact was needed to cause the injuries.

1. The defense risks juries finding that the defendants caused severe impact as well as violent and sustained shaking.

2. Prosecutors must refute any claim that impact is required *and* that if impact was sufficient to cause death, it *must* be accompanied by skull fracture, neck injury, or other external marks of impact injury.

— Defense medical experts discuss each injury as though it occurred in isolation.

1. Compel defense experts to consider all the child's injuries together.

2. When classic findings of AHT are considered together, no other medical condition fully mimics the result.[10]

— Some defense medical experts offer theories without scientific merit.

1. Consider a pretrial motion hearing to explore the scientific basis of opinions.

2. Put the claim in accurate epidemiological context.

3. Judge each case on the nature of the fall, the acceleration-deceleration forces involved, and the location and nature of the head injury.

4. Acknowledge case-law limitations on admissibility of scientific evidence. The US Supreme Court's decision in *Daubert v Merrell Dow Pharmaceuticals* provides a useful test for the reliability of theories of causation.[11]

   A. Trial court judges must review expert testimony and allow into evidence only opinions reliable enough to help the jury.

   B. Medical witnesses should have experience working with pediatric patients or child victims of homicide, undergo training to update expertise, and have trained others and/or contributed to the medical literature in the field.

REBUTTAL WITNESSES
— Call or re-call expert witnesses to rebut defense theories.

— Never assume jurors or judges understand weaknesses in the defense experts' testimony without the assistance of rebuttal experts.

— Obtain the judge's permission in advance to have the prosecution's experts listen to defense experts' testimony and extend the same courtesy to defense experts.

— Keep everything concise, simple, and clear.

1. Only cover points addressed by defense witnesses.

2. Put testimony in proper scientific perspective according to case facts.

3. Clarify:

    A. That the injuries are consistent solely with having been inflicted.

    B. There is no lucid interval in children with massive brain injuries.

    C. Young children are not strong enough to cause diffuse brain injuries in infants.

    D. Injuries consistent with short falls differ from those seen in violent shaking or massive head impacts.

PERSUASION IN THE COURTROOM

OPENING STATEMENT

— Choose a theme for the case based on the evidence. Include information about the child, the child's relationship with the defendant, the nature of the injuries, the mechanism needed to explain the injuries, the outcome for the victim, and the victim's innocence with respect to the outcome.

— Do not argue the case in the opening statement.

— Help jurors understand what the crime entails.

1. Define the crime as a violent assault against a child who was depending on the defendant for safety, support, and sustenance.

2. Focus on the victim as a real person—a child.

— Message to jurors:

1. Be prepared to keep an open mind.

2. Understand that injury pictures will be disturbing.

3. See injuries as the only way the victim can express what happened.

4. Summarize the evidence.

5. Alert jurors that each witness offers 1 piece of the picture and they need to piece it together and reach a conclusion.

Personalizing the Victim
— Always use the victim's name and instruct witnesses to use it during testimony.

— Introduce videotapes or photographs of moments in the victim's life before injury.

— Remind jurors of what was known about the child during the child's short life.

Closing Argument
— In serious child abuse and homicide cases, the closing argument may be more important than in many other types of criminal prosecutions.

— Requires advance preparation and adaptation during trial as evidence is introduced.

— Summarize what happened to the victim, what type of assault was involved, how injuries were caused, and who committed the acts.

— Emphasize the strength of the medical evidence and convince jurors that violent assault is the only possibility and the defendant is the only possible perpetrator.

— Remind jurors there is no profile of a typical child abuser.

— Repeat expert testimony that anyone who becomes stressed during childcare is capable of violence.

— Use visual aids to make critical points.

— Acknowledge the difficult job of sitting in judgment of the actions of another person.

1. Simplify legal elements of criminal statutes to make explanations consistent with the law, yet understandable to laypersons.

2. Reassure the jury that the state's lawmakers labeled those who commit the crime as criminals/murderers, and jurors simply judge whether the facts of the case fit the legal elements of the crime.

— Focus on tragedy of child murder.

— Emphasize that stress is not a mitigating factor.

— Leave a final image: the perspective of the victim during the moments preceding the final, fatal act of abuse.

REFERENCES

1. National Center for Prosecution of Child Abuse. *Manual on Investigation and Prosecution of Child Abuse.* 2nd ed. Alexandria, Va: American Prosecutors Research Institute; 1993.

2. *State v Mott*, 931 P2d 1046 (Ariz 1997).

3. Fed R Evid 703.

4. Laridson J, Parrish R. Computer graphics in child abuse and neglect. *APSAC Advisor.* 2001;13:14-18.

5. *People v Hood*, 53 Cal App 4th 965, 62 Cal Rptr 2d 137 (1997).

6. *State v Bluff*, 52 P3d 1210 (Utah 2002).

7. Alexander RC, Smith WL. Shaken baby syndrome. *Infants Young Child.* 1998;10:1-9.

8. Feldman KW. Evaluation of physical abuse. In: Helfer ME, Kempe RS, Krugman RD, eds. *The Battered Child.* 5th ed. Chicago, Ill: University of Chicago Press; 1997:175-220.

9. Fed R Evid 404, 405.

10. Duhaime AC, Christian CW, Rorke LB, Zimmerman RA. Non-accidental head injury in infants—the "shaken baby syndrome." *N Engl J Med.* 1998;338:1822-1829.

11. *Daubert v Merrell Dow Pharmaceuticals, Inc*, 509 US 579 (1993).

Chapter 13

NEURODEVELOPMENTAL OUTCOMES OF ABUSIVE HEAD TRAUMA

Karen Kirhofer-Hansen, MD
Gary L. Hedlund, DO
Deborah E. Lowen, MD

— The prognosis includes risk of death in the acute phase and the possibility of long-term neurological damage if the child survives.

— The outcome of abusive head trauma (AHT) affects the child's quality of life, medical care, rehabilitation, placement, and prosecution.

FACTORS INFLUENCING OUTCOME

— Often, caregivers do not provide accurate histories in AHT cases.

— There is a high likelihood that AHT is not accurately diagnosed when victims are younger, of low socioeconomic status, and/or have less severe symptoms.

— It is possible that victims were subjected to more than 1 episode of head trauma, making outcome assessment more complex.

— Mechanisms of injury:

1. Include contact, acceleration-deceleration, or hypoxia-ischemia.[1]

2. Can occur alone or in combination.

3. Some mechanisms do not cause clinically evident injury acutely.

— A child may be injured even though continual developmental progress is normal.

1. Evaluating outcome at a single point in time may be inadequate. Longitudinal assessment is necessary.

2. Access to the child can be complicated by out-of-home placement, confidentiality issues, and lack of cooperation by nonoffending family members who do not believe the child suffered AHT.

MORBIDITY

OUTCOME ASSESSMENT

— An outcome assessment can be a simple description such as "survived" or "did not survive," or a detailed analysis of specific sensorimotor, cognitive, or behavioral problems.

— No single test meets all desirable criteria.

— Outcome measures include clinical judgments, psychometric tests, and rating scales and interviews.[2]

Clinical Judgments

— Are based on medical record review or the Glasgow Outcome Scale,[3] which assigns an ordinal value to the qualitative assessment of the degree of disability.

— The subjective nature and lack of sensitivity to subtle deficits are drawbacks.

Psychometric Tests

— Provide quantitative data and are often given by neuropsychologists or developmental specialists.

— These tests may not assess social competence, behavioral adjustment, adaptive functioning, etc.[4]

Rating Scales and Interviews

— Address the weaknesses of psychometric tests and include the Vineland Adaptive Behavior Scales,[5] the Child Behavior Checklist,[6] and the Functional Independence Measure for Children (WeeFIM).[7]

— The information is highly dependent on the source, and some rating scales are not appropriate for use with head-injured children or not sensitive enough to detect problems.[4]

INFORMATION SOURCES
— There is scant medical literature on outcomes after AHT.

— Outcomes after pediatric head trauma do not clearly extrapolate to AHT cases because of differences in:

1. Mechanisms of injury.

2. Clinical, radiographic, and pathologic findings.

3. Effects on ultimate neurodevelopmental outcomes.

— Sample populations studied:

1. Young children are the primary victims of abusive head injuries; most victims are younger than 12 months.

2. Most pediatric head trauma research excludes infants and very young children, groups them with older children, or has an insufficient sample size of young children.

AGE AT INJURY
— Younger infants may benefit from the plasticity of the brain and greater recuperative abilities.

— Irreparable disruption in the ordered sequence of neurological development can occur; certain skills are especially vulnerable.

— The literature is unclear on the effect of age on later outcomes.[8]

— Injuries sustained by infants and very young children are associated with more deficits than injuries sustained by preschool-aged or older children.[4]

— Greater neurological damage can result from the size difference between perpetrators and infants.

— A younger infant's exposure to rotational forces is greater due to a larger head size relative to neck musculature.

— Difference in myelination causes greater susceptibility to cerebral damage.

SEVERITY OF ACUTE INJURY
— More severe initial injuries produce worse outcomes.

1. Severity of injury is usually measured in terms of neurological impairment.

2. Severity is assessed by length of impaired consciousness, duration of posttraumatic amnesia, or formal scales such as the Glasgow Coma Scale.[9]

— AHT victims can initially have relatively mild symptoms that do not correlate with the severity of the underlying brain injury or predict better outcome.

RADIOGRAPHIC FINDINGS

— Severity of pathology on cranial imaging correlates with outcome in patients of different ages regardless of injury mechanism.

— Findings on initial computed tomography (CT) scans of patients with subdural hematomas that correlate with worse outcomes (**Figures 13-1-a** and **b**) include basal cistern compression or absence, significant subarachnoid hemorrhage, midline shift, and intraventricular hemorrhage.[10]

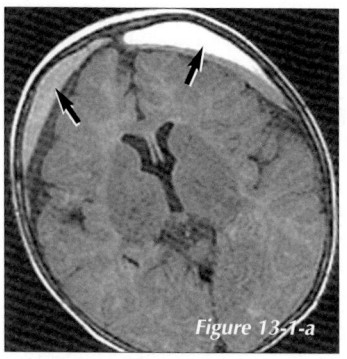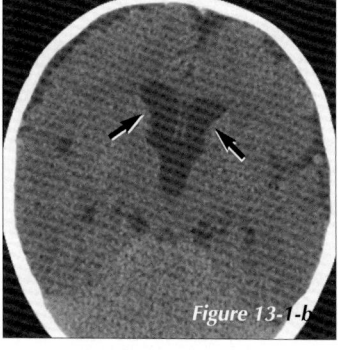

Figure 13-1-a

Figure 13-1-b

Figure 13-1-a. Axial fluid attenuating inversion recovery MRI scan of 6-month-old boy with increasing head circumference demonstrates increased signal intensity of chronic bilateral subdural collections of varying ages in the frontotemporal area (arrows).

Figure 13-1-b. Same child as in 13-1-a. Axial noncontrast CT image taken 4 months later shows resolution of subdural hematomas. Frontal horns (arrows) and third ventricle dilated, probably related to obstructive hydrocephalus. Brain appears normal.

— Presence of parenchymal damage:

1. The initial CT scan may underestimate injury, so closely assess the "worst" CT scan.[11]

2. This damage is more likely to cause coagulation defects and produce worse outcomes.

— Other prognostic factors:

1. Edema.[12-17] Cranial imaging evidence of severe cerebral edema portends severe neurological impairment.[13]

2. Overall, diffuse brain swelling results in greater morbidity than focal swelling.

— Posttraumatic infarction is common after accidental and inflicted traumatic brain injury.[14,18]

1. Recognition is limited by the type and timing of cranial imaging.

2. Diffusion-weighted imaging (DWI) with magnetic resonance imaging (MRI):

    A. It is more sensitive than CT or conventional MRI to detect posttraumatic ischemia, especially in young children with incomplete myelinization.

    B. Severity of injury detected by DWI is significantly associated with outcome at hospital discharge.

— Diffuse axonal injury:

1. Was originally a neuropathologic diagnosis in victims of traumatic brain injury who suffered prolonged coma and had microscopic damage to cerebral white matter at autopsy.

2. Is also termed traumatic axonal injury (white-matter shearing tears).

3. Is best detected with specific MRI techniques, but CT or ultrasound is also useful.[10]

4. Diagnosis indicates severe brain damage with very poor outcomes.

5. Some cases, especially focal, are undetected clinically, radiographically, or pathologically.

6. Cerebral atrophy can be found on cranial imaging studies and by significant decrease in the rate of head circumference growth (microcephaly).

7. May be unable to differentiate atrophy caused by traumatic injury from that caused by severe hypoxia-ischemia.[10]

8. This injury is associated with more severe neurological sequelae in AHT victims.[19-21]

LABORATORY VALUES

— Hyperglycemia at admission is closely related to severity of injury.[16,22]

— Elevated blood glucose level is significantly associated with poorer outcome on the Glasgow Outcome Scale.[16,23,24]

— Children with initial blood glucose levels greater than 200 mg/dL have worse outcomes.

— Coagulopathy complicates traumatic brain injury in AHT victims.[25]

— Disseminated intravascular coagulation is associated with greater morbidity and mortality.[16,26,27]

NEUROLOGICAL SIGNS

— Children and adults with closed head injuries are at risk for elevated intracranial pressure (ICP), possibly causing brain herniation and death.

— In AHT, elevated ICP is more often caused by brain swelling.

— Early posttraumatic seizures (EPTS):

1. Seizures occurring within 1 week of injury,[28] seen in both adult and pediatric patients with head injuries

2. Correlation between severity of injury and occurrence of EPTS[16]:

   A. EPTS influences outcomes by causing secondary brain injuries, especially if hypoxia occurs during the seizures.

   B. The incidence of EPTS with AHT is higher than with accidental head trauma.

— Severe acute brain injury causes EPTS, posttraumatic epilepsy, and poor outcome.

RETINAL FINDINGS

— Retinal hemorrhages are not associated with later visual loss.

— Optic nerve atrophy contributes to long-term vision loss, possibly because of direct optic nerve injury.[29]

LATER FINDINGS

MICROCEPHALY AND CEREBRAL ATROPHY

— Impaired head growth and resultant microcephaly in AHT results from cerebral atrophy and portends significant long-term neurological impairment.

— Survivors of AHT require close monitoring for cerebral atrophy and microcephaly. The prognosis is modified as needed.

POSTTRAUMATIC EPILEPSY

— Occurs in about 2% of survivors of pediatric head trauma, about 10% of children with penetrating injury or depressed skull fractures,[4] and 20% to 50% of AHT victims.[14,15,20,30]

— Posttraumatic epilepsy itself may contribute to greater morbidity, but it more likely signals greater neurological derangement.

SPECIFIC NEURODEVELOPMENTAL DELAYS

— Delays in cognitive, motor, and behavioral development are common in survivors of pediatric head trauma in general and AHT in particular (**Figures 13-2-a, b,** and **c**).

Cognitive Status

— Cognitive impairment in school-aged children is usually measured with intelligence tests.

1. Deficits are common after accidental head injury, with the degree of deficit related to injury severity.[4]

2. Children often recover some intellectual function in the immediate postinjury phase, but IQ scores remain lower than preinjury levels.[31,32]

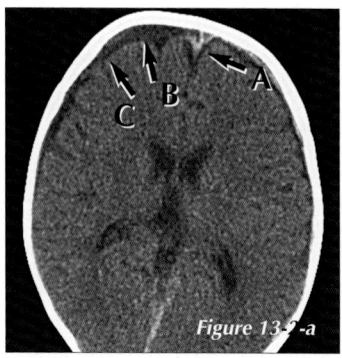

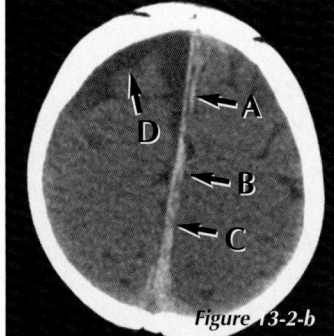

Figures 13-2-a and **b.** Axial noncontrast CT images of 17-month-old girl with severe intellectual delay and cognitive impairment.

Figure 13-2-a. Acute anterior inter-hemispheric parafalcine subdural hemorrhage (arrow A). Also note a chronic small right frontotemporal subdural collection (arrows B and C).

Figure 13-2-b. Scan through cerebral convexity shows acute left parafalcine subdural hemorrhage (arrows A, B, and C) and a chronic right frontal subdural hematoma (arrow D).

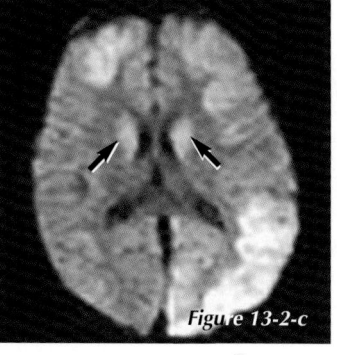

Figure 13-2-c. Axial diffusion MRI scan. Multifocal regions of diffusion restriction indicate cerebral infarction, including bilateral frontal lobes and caudate nuclei (arrows). The left hemisphere is more severely involved.

— Infants and very young children with AHT injuries have lower cognitive scores than expected based on injury severity alone.[33]

— The difference in cognitive scores between abused and accidentally injured children persists.[17,33]

— Limited repertoire of cognitive skills may obscure true deficit.

— Problems are revealed as age-appropriate development fails to occur.

Motor Status

— In accidental traumatic brain injury, motor deficits depend on the severity and specific location of injury in the brain.

— Motor scores in children with severe accidental head injuries are lower than IQ scores,[8] especially in children with cerebral edema or infarctions.[17]

— Motor problems are seen in up to 80% of AHT survivors.[14,20]

Behavior

— Emotional and behavioral issues are common in victims of pediatric head trauma.

— Symptoms range from mild difficulties with moodiness and impulsivity to attention deficit hyperactivity disorder, anxiety disorder, and depression.[34,35]

— Injury severity correlates with resulting emotional and behavioral abnormalities.

— In school-aged children, emotional and behavioral difficulties are related to both brain trauma and parent and family risk factors.[36]

— Symptoms increase during the first year after injury.

— The family of a child with severe traumatic brain injury has a high level of family burden and stress in the immediate postinjury phase and 1 year later.[37]

— The child's emotional and behavioral issues contribute to family stress, which contributes to greater emotional and behavioral problems in the child.[38]

— Evaluation of infants and very young children for emotional and behavioral problems focuses primarily on cognitive and motor outcomes.

— AHT victims manifest behavioral and emotional problems in the immediate postinjury phase and over time.

— These problems may be inadequately addressed by medical providers or school environments.

Effects of Delays

— Disabilities associated with deficits limit daily functioning.

— The children become familial and societal burdens in terms of personnel and financial resources (**Figures 13-3-a** and **b**).

— Delayed recognition of deficits is common in AHT victims because of difficulty testing, lack of personnel and reimbursement for testing, and inadequate follow-up.

— Close follow-up shows many AHT victims have sequelae.[20,39]

— The "sign-free" interval illustrates the importance of close follow-up to identify disabilities and provide rehabilitation services.

— Medical providers must explain status to give parents and caregivers realistic expectations.

— Child protection, law enforcement, and prosecution officials must understand that if a child appears "normal" in the first few months after AHT, it neither diminishes the crime's severity nor implies the child will be unaffected.

FACTORS THAT MODERATE OUTCOMES

— Preinjury and postinjury family environment, especially regarding emotional and behavioral outcomes[32,40]

— Family functioning at the time of acute injuries

— Provision of resources to families

MORTALITY

FACTORS COMPLICATING ACCURATE DETERMINATION

— Differing mechanisms of injury

— Inadequate histories, and therefore lack of appropriate diagnosis

— Lack of long-term follow-up to document deaths occurring later; often exclude children who die before receiving medical care

— Lack of data on withdrawal of medical support from severely impaired children

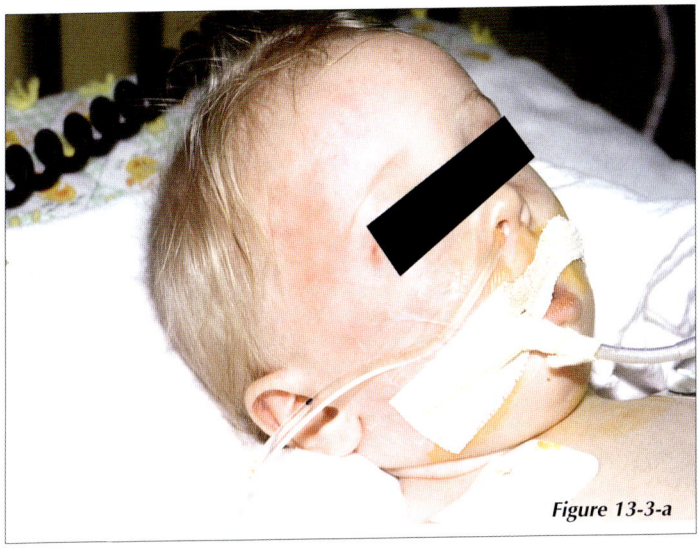

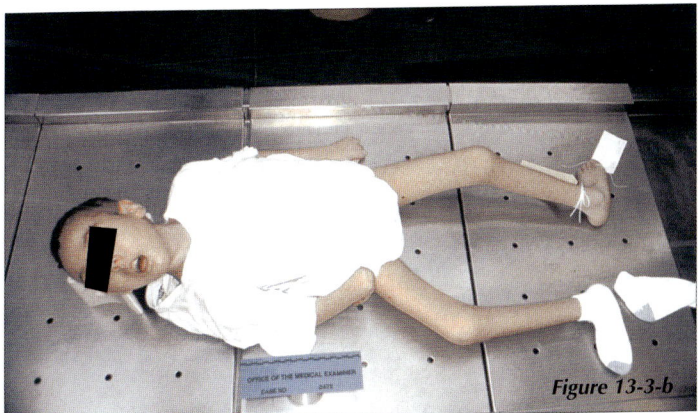

Figure 13-3-a. *Extensive bruising of face and ear consistent with slap or multiple impacts to side of 6-month-old boy's face.*

Figure 13-3-b. *Autopsy photo shows severely impaired 12½-year-old boy. Note emaciation and musculoskeletal contractures.*

— Shaken children, with or without impact, demonstrate brain injury in the majority of fatalities. The usual cause of injury/death is uncontrollable intracranial hypertension resulting from cerebral edema (**Figures 13-4-a, b,** and **c**).

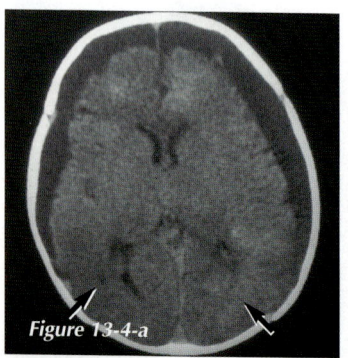 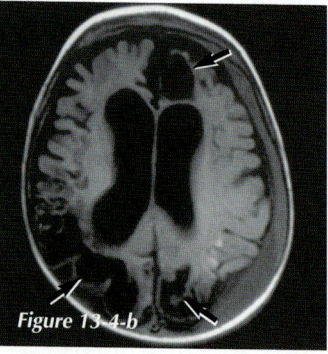

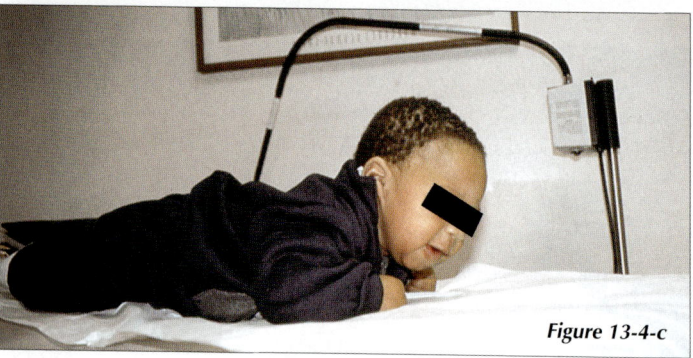

Figure 13-4-a. Axial noncontrast CT image of 1-month-old boy shows occipital lobe edema (arrows) and chronic bilateral subdural hematomas.

Figure 13-4-b. Axial T1-weighted MRI scan taken 6 months later. Note diffuse cerebral hemispheric atrophy, cystic encephalomalacia prominent at sites of original edema (arrows) and chronic left subdural hematoma.

Figure 13-4-c. At age 2 years, the boy has severe neurological impairment reflected in small size, body position, and general appearance.

REFERENCES

1. Alexander R, Crabbe L, Sato Y, Smith W, Bennett T. Serial abuse in children who are shaken. *Am J Dis Child*. 1990;144:58-60.

2. Fletcher JM, Ewing-Cobbs L, Francis DJ, Levin HS. Variability in outcomes after traumatic brain injury in children: a developmental perspective. In: Broman SH, Michel ME. eds. *Traumatic Head Injury in Children*. New York, NY: Oxford University Press; 1995: 3-21.

3. Jennett B, Bond M. Assessment of outcome after severe brain damage. *Lancet*. 1975;1:480-484.

4. Yeates KO. Closed-head injury. In: Yeates KO, Ris MD, Taylor HG, eds. *Pediatric Neuropsychology: Research, Theory, and Practice*. New York, NY: Guilford Press; 2000:92-116.

5. Sparrow SS, Balla DA, Cicchetti DV. *Vineland Adaptive Behavior Scales*. Circle Pines, Minn: American Guidance Service; 1984.

6. Achenbach TM. *Manual for the Child Behavior Checklist/4-18 and 1991 Profile*. Burlington: Department of Psychiatry, University of Vermont; 1991.

7. *Guide for the use of the Uniform Data System for Medical Rehabilitation, including the Functional Independence Measure for Children (WeeFIM). Version 1.5*. Buffalo: State University of New York at Buffalo; 1991.

8. Ewing-Cobbs L, Fletcher JM, Levin HS, Francis DJ, Davidson K, Miner ME. Longitudinal neuropsychological outcome in infants and preschoolers with traumatic brain injury. *J Int Neuropsychol Soc*. 1997;3:581-591.

9. Teasdale G, Jennett B. Assessment of coma and impaired consciousness. A practical scale. *Lancet*. 1974;2:81-84.

10. Kleinman PK, Barnes PD. Head trauma. In: Kleinman PK, ed. *Diagnostic Imaging of Child Abuse*. 2nd ed. St Louis, Mo: Mosby; 1998;285-342.

11. Servadei F, Nasi M, Giuliani G, et al. CT prognostic factors in acute subdural haematomas: the value of the 'worst' CT scan. *Br J Neurosurg.* 2000;14:110-116.

12. Ewing-Cobbs L, Kramer L, Prasad M, et al. Neuroimaging, physical, and developmental findings after inflicted and noninflicted traumatic brain injury in young children. *Pediatrics.* 1998;102:300-307.

13. Duhaime AC, Christian C, Moss E, Seidl T. Long-term outcome in infants with the shaking-impact syndrome. *Pediatr Neurosurg.* 1996;24:292-300.

14. Gilles E, Nelson MD Jr. Cerebral complications of nonaccidental head injury in childhood. *Pediatr Neurol.* 1998;19:119-128.

15. Hirsch W, Schobess A, Eichler G, Zumkeller W, Teichler H, Schluter A. Severe head trauma in children: cranial computer tomography and clinical consequences. *Paediatr Anaesth.* 2002;12:337-344.

16. Chiaretti A, Piastra M, Pulitano S, et al. Prognostic factors and outcome of children with severe head injury: an 8-year experience. *Childs Nerv Syst.* 2002;18:129-136.

17. Ewing-Cobbs L, Prasad M, Kramer L, Landry S. Inflicted traumatic brain injury: relationship of developmental outcome to severity of injury. *Pediatr Neurosurg.* 1999;31:251-258.

18. Server A, Dullerud R, Haakonsen M, Nakstad PH, Johnsen UL, Magnaes B. Post-traumatic cerebral infarction. Neuroimaging findings, etiology and outcome. *Acta Radiol.* 2001;42:254-260.

19. Sinal SH, Ball MR. Head trauma due to child abuse: serial computerized tomography in diagnosis and management. *South Med J.* 1987;80:1505-1512.

20. Bonnier C, Nassogne MC, Evrard P. Outcome and prognosis of whiplash shaken infant syndrome; late consequences after a symptom-free interval. *Dev Med Child Neurol.* 1995;37:943-956.

21. Ludwig S, Warman M. Shaken baby syndrome: a review of 20 cases. *Ann Emerg Med*. 1984;13:104-107.

22. Lam AM, Winn HR, Cullen BF, Sundling N. Hyperglycaemia and neurological outcome in patients with head injury. *J Neurosurg*. 1991;75:545-551.

23. Michaud LJ, Rivara FP, Longstreth WT Jr, Grady MS. Elevated initial blood glucose levels and poor outcome following severe brain injuries in children. *J Trauma*. 1991;31:1356-1362.

24. Chiaretti A, De Benedictis R, Langer A, et al. Prognostic implications of hyperglycaemia in paediatric head injury. *Childs Nerv Syst*. 1998;14:455-459.

25. Hymel KP, Abshire TC, Luckey DW, Jenny C. Coagulopathy in pediatric abusive head trauma. *Pediatrics*. 1997;99:371-375.

26. Vavilala MS, Dunbar PJ, Rivara FP, Lam AM. Coagulopathy predicts poor outcome following head injury in children less than 16 years of age. *J Neurosurg Anesthesiol*. 2001;13:13-18.

27. Becker S, Schneider W, Kreuz W, Jacobi G, Scharrer I, Nowak-Gottl U. Post-trauma coagulation and fibrinolysis in children suffering from severe cerebrocranial trauma. *Eur J Pediatr*. 1999;158 (suppl):197-202.

28. Jennett B. Trauma as a cause of epilepsy in childhood. *Dev Med Child Neurol*. 1973;15:56-62.

29. Levin AV. Retinal hemorrhages and child abuse. In: David TJ, ed. *Recent Advances of Paediatrics*. Vol 18. Edinburgh, Scotland: Churchill Livingstone; 2000:151-219.

30. Jayawant S, Rawlinson A, Gibbon F, et al. Subdural haemorrhages in infants: population based study. *BMJ*. 1998;317:1558-1561.

31. Klonoff H, Clark C, Klonoff PS. Long-term outcome of head injuries: a 23 year follow up study of children with head injuries. *J Neurol Neurosurg Psychiatry*. 1993;56:410-415.

32. Yeates KO, Wade Sl, Stancin T, Taylor HG, Drotar D, Minich N. A prospective study of short- and long-term neuropsychological outcomes after traumatic brain injury in children. *Neuropsychology*. 2002;16:514-523.

33. Prasad M, Ewing-Cobbs L, Swank P, Kramer L. Predictors of outcome following traumatic brain injury in young children. *Pediatr Neurosurg*. 2002;36:64-74.

34. Shaffer D. Behavioral sequelae of serious head injury in children and adolescents: the British studies. In: Broman SH, Michel ME, eds. *Traumatic Head Injury in Children*. New York, NY: Oxford University Press; 1995:55-69.

35. Luis CA, Mittenberg W. Mood and anxiety disorders following pediatric traumatic brain injury: a prospective study. *J Clin Exp Neuropsychol*. 2002;24:270-279.

36. Yeates K, Taylor H, Barry C, Drotar D, Wade S, Stancin T. Neurobehavioral symptoms in childhood closed-head injuries: changes in prevalence and correlates during the first year postinjury. *J Pediatr Psychol*. 2001;26:79-91.

37. Wade Wl, Taylor HG, Drotar D, Stancin T, Yeates KO. Family burden and adaptation during the initial year after traumatic brain injury in children. *Pediatrics*. 1998;102(pt 1):110-116.

38. Taylor HG, Yeates KO, Wade SL, Drotar D, Stancin T, Burant C. Bidirectional child-family influences on outcomes of traumatic brain injury in children. *J Int Neuropsychol Soc*. 2001;7:755-767.

39. Fischer H, Allasio D. Permanently damaged: long-term follow-up of shaken babies. *Clin Pediatr (Phila)*. 1994;33:696-698.

40. Yeates KO, Taylor HG, Drotar D, et al. Preinjury family environment as a determinant of recovery from traumatic brain injuries in school-age children. *J Int Neuropsychol Soc*. 1997;3:617-630.

Chapter 14

PREVENTION AND EDUCATION

Marilyn Barr, BIS, SSW
Ronald Barr, MDCM, FRCPC
Trina Taylor, BS, SSW
Amy Wicks
Deborah Williams, BIS
Karen Coleman

— Continuous education about the dangers of shaking young children is necessary.

— Identify victim and perpetrator characteristics to direct future education and prevention efforts (**Figure 14-1**).

— Review the National Center on Shaken Baby Syndrome's (NCSBS) database of victims of shaken baby syndrome (SBS) cases reported since 1978.

1. The database includes victim and perpetrator profiles, medical findings, charges filed, and court outcomes when available.

2. Details help identify trends and improve targeting of prevention programs.

TARGETED PROGRAMS

OFFENDER PROFILE

— Men outnumber women in every known study of SBS offenders.

— The perpetrator most likely to confess to shaking an infant is the biological father.

TRIGGERS

— Inconsolable crying

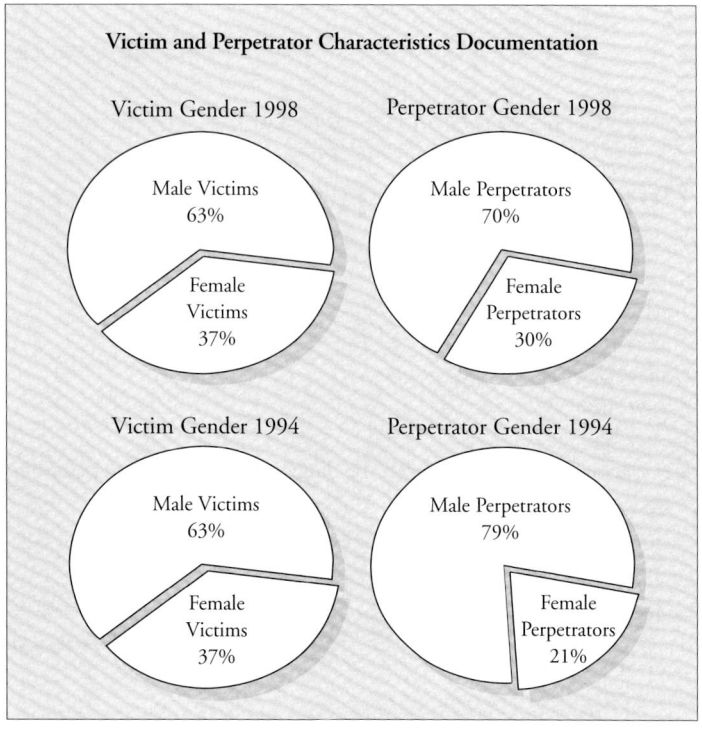

Figure 14-1. *Breakdown of child abuse victims and perpetrators by gender. Adapted from the NCSBS.*[1]

— Stimuli in conflict with caregiver expectations and beyond caregiver control

TOPICS TO ADDRESS

— What to do when confronted with an apparently inconsolable infant

— How to handle toddlers during temper tantrums

— How to walk away and regain composure rather than lose emotional control and harm the infant through anger or frustration

— Crying

Facts About Crying

— Pediatricians should ask parents about their response to a crying infant as part of anticipatory guidance to prevent SBS.

1. Crying in normal infants has a robust, well-established pattern often referred to as the normal crying curve.

2. The number of hours of crying per day increases at about age 2 weeks, rises to a peak during the second month of life, and then decreases to stable lower levels by about the fourth month.[2,3]

3. Other characteristics causing frustration include crying episodes lasting 40 minutes (on average), crying bouts resistant to soothing, and clustering of crying during late afternoon and evening hours.[4]

4. Clinical cases of SBS are more likely to occur with a similar pattern to the ages when these frustrating crying characteristics occur.

— Caregivers need information on crying in normal infants and how and when to ask for help or emotional support.

— Caregivers also need to be empowered to seek help and assured that admitting the need for a break and asking for help do not indicate failure as a caregiver.

Avoiding Misinformation

— Scare tactics and misinformation can create unjustified fear in parents about harming their infants.

— Juries and judges can be led to believe it is easy to cause SBS.

— It takes an extremely violent assault to produce life-threatening injuries. Brain damage is not caused by normal caregiving activities.

Target Audiences

— Men and boys. Reach them through prenatal classes, schools, colleges, training for early childhood educators, correctional facilities, military bases, and television programs directed toward men.

— Childcare providers

1. Reach them through SBS prevention groups and childcare licensing and training agencies.

2. Legislation and policies mandate such training.[5]

— New parents

1. Often, they have unrealistic expectations and heightened levels of frustration.

2. Reach them through prenatal and postnatal classes and hospital-based prevention programs.

3. It is a challenge to reach those dealing with an inconsolable crying infant or an infant who has colic. The goal is to help them understand how to deal with their frustration and give them a sense of competence through education on crying issues.

— Young people before they become parents. Reach them through community youth and religious groups as well as during school as part of health or lifestyle courses.

— Mothers

1. Mothers are the most likely to care for and be alone with infants for long periods of time.

2. They are the most efficient conduits for educating those who are the most common perpetrators (husbands, partners, or others who care for their children).

3. They have a vested interest in the welfare of their infants and are likely to take on the role of protecting their children.

— Medical personnel

1. Prevention requires familiarity with the signs and symptoms of SBS and how to properly diagnose the syndrome.

2. They need education on the normal crying curve and crying-related behaviors.

3. They should be familiar with local resources offering respite for stressed caregivers, as respite is important to prevention.

4. Crisis nurseries, community parent groups that provide information and support, and family, friends, and professional childcare workers can help parents at stressful times.

PROGRAMS FOR FATHERS, EXPECTANT FATHERS, AND OTHER MEN

— Educate men about the dangers of shaking, help them learn infant care skills, and encourage discussion about their perceptions of fatherhood.

— Include the latest SBS research, with data on injuries caused by shaking, factors that may trigger shaking, and demographics of victim and perpetrator profiles.

— Give new fathers accurate information about crying behavior, which may help them develop age-appropriate expectations for their infants.

— Teach them how to deal with inconsolable crying and how to recognize crying patterns.

— "Dads 101," a course made available through the NCSBS, is designed for fathers and male caregivers.

1. The course provides the opportunity for men to learn basic parenting skills.

2. It is designed specifically for men going through pregnancy with their partners.

3. It is taught by fathers.

4. It gives them the opportunity to talk about their greatest fears and concerns regarding fatherhood.

5. It allows fathers to discuss their preparations for fatherhood, the changes their partners experience during pregnancy, and their long-term hopes and fears about being fathers.

6. It gives men the chance to ask questions about pregnancy, delivery, and childcare that they may not feel comfortable asking their partners or physicians.

7. Practicing the basics of infant care helps fathers gain confidence and feel more prepared.

8. Topics such as how to deal with an inconsolable crying infant, how to ask for help, and the dangers of shaking an infant are discussed.

PROGRAMS ON INFANT CRYING

— *The Period of PURPLE Crying* aims to prevent SBS through education about normal, but frustrating behavior linked to shaking.

— Each letter of PURPLE refers to 1 of the 6 most common and most frustrating characteristics of crying (**Table 14-1**).

— The program includes a booklet and companion film designed to increase knowledge and change behaviors of parents and to provide healthcare practitioners with resources on infant crying, thus reducing the incidence of abuse.

Table 14-1. The Period of PURPLE Crying

PEAK PATTERN

The total amount of daily distress behavior (fussing, crying, and/or "colic" crying) tends to increase into the second month of age and then decrease, independent of caregiving style or the parents' abilities.

UNPREDICTABLE

Crying bouts seem to start and stop with no apparent relationship to anything happening in the environment, and therefore appear spontaneous and unexplained.

RESISTANT TO SOOTHING

One of the most frustrating characteristics of early infant crying, infants become inconsolable when crying.

PAIN-LIKE FACE

Infants appear to be in pain, which increases the anxiety and stress of caregivers. However, healthy, crying infants can look like they are in pain even when they may not be.

(continued)

> **Table 14-1.** *(continued)*
>
> LONG CRYING BOUTS
>
> Infants can have crying bouts that persist from a few minutes to 1 or 2 hours. These prolonged periods of crying are typical only in the first 3 or 4 months of life, and rarely occur later. However, the crying causes distress and frustration for caregivers.
>
> EVENING CRYING
>
> Crying tends to be clustered in the late afternoon and evening, especially in the first few months of life.
>
> *Adapted from Barr,[2,3] and Barr et al.[4,6]*

HOSPITAL-BASED PROGRAMS FOR NEW PARENTS

— Parents receive instructions before leaving the hospital with their newborn.

— Parents are warned against shaking their infants and instructed on how to cope with crying infants.

— The programs illustrate how fatigue and frustration can lead to shaking an infant.

— Nurses are encouraged to teach the program.

— Instruction is given separately from all other information.

— The programs include verbal, written, and visual instruction.

1. Written materials include cards, pamphlets, or booklets.

2. Visual reminders include magnets, bookmarks, or posters with the message never to shake an infant.

    A. The reminders can evoke emotional responses to reinforce the concept that parents are their children's best advocates.

    B. The reminders underscore the importance of parents teaching others who care for their infants about the harmful effects of shaking.

— Commitment statement:

1. Parents are asked to complete and sign a commitment statement that requests basic demographic information.

2. By signing the statement, the parents acknowledge they have received information on SBS and will educate others who care for their child.

3. The statement requests permission to contact the parents for a follow-up call 6 to 7 months after the birth of their child.

4. In the follow-up call, parents are asked if they remember receiving information on SBS and what they remember most.

5. They may also be asked to indicate a contact person if they become frustrated with the child and feel that they need help.

6. The process establishes a plan of action parents can activate should the need arise.

SCHOOL-BASED PROGRAMS FOR YOUTHS

— In classroom settings, educators have regular access to students throughout their developmental years.

— The setting and time of the program as well as the target audience and program content must be considered.

— Include information on infant development, reasonable expec-tations about caring for infants, SBS and the physical outcomes of shaking an infant, activities in which students can discuss how to care for an incon-solable infant and how and when to get help, and films about SBS cases.

— Family members of victims of SBS may attend class and share their stories.

— At least 2 hours are required to briefly discuss all topics and show a film.

— Ideally, the program should be provided for an individual class, or no more than 30 students, rather than a large auditorium in order to encourage student interaction.

— Many concepts are too complex for younger children; consider the maturity of the students.

— Topics for school-based programs:

1. Perception and definition of gender roles and stereotypes

2. Realistic expectations

3. Coping with crying

4. Prevention planning

5. Explanation and dynamics of SBS

TRAINING FOR CHILDCARE PROVIDERS

— Require training on the dangers of shaking infants as well as what instigates shaking.

— Childcare providers are continuously faced with fussy infants and inconsolable crying, which may lead to shaking.

— Teach providers to form relationships with the children and their parents, giving them an opportunity to watch for signs of abuse and educate the parents.

OTHER ACTIVITIES AND PUBLIC EDUCATION

— Family members of victims have become strong advocates for change.

— Many states have laws requiring hospitals, school classrooms, and daycare centers to provide SBS education.

— Include:

1. Posters

2. Printed materials about crying

3. Information for fathers

4. Educational videos and documentaries

5. Computer graphics and animations

FUNDING

— Prevention is likely to be cost-effective.

— Requires creative and innovative methods to raise support.

— Sources may include children's trust funds, private foundations, donors, and government grants.

— Can involve private health care insurers, Medicaid, and public agencies.

— May occur through donations or as part of pay-for-service arrangements.

REFERENCES

1. National Center on Shaken Baby Syndrome. *Dads 101: A Training Program for New and Expectant Fathers.* Ogden, Utah: National Center on Shaken Baby Syndrome; 2002.

2. Barr RG. The normal crying curve: what do we really know? *Dev Med Child Neurol.* 1990;32:356-362.

3. Barr RG. Excessive crying. In: Sameroff AJ, Lewis M, Miller SM, eds. *Handbook of Developmental Psychopathology.* 2nd ed. New York, NY: Springer; 2000:327-350.

4. Barr RG, Paterson JA, MacMartin LM, Lehtonen L, Young SN. Prolonged and unsoothable crying bouts in infants with and without colic. *J Dev Behav Pediatr.* 2005;26:14-23.

5. Legislation. National Center on Shaken Baby Syndrome Web site. Available at: http://www.dontshake.com/Subject.aspx?categoryID= 5&PageName-FutEffortLegislation.htm. Accessed October 21, 2005.

6. Barr RG, Trent RB, Cross J. Age-related incidence curve of hospitalized shaken baby syndrome cases: convergent evidence for crying as a trigger to shaking. *Child Abuse Negl.* 2006;30:7-16.

INDEX

A

Abdomen, objective assessment, 18
Abdominal bruising, 126f
Abdominal injuries, 124t
Abdominal trauma, 123-127
Abuse
    commitment, establishment, 261
    confession, investigation continuation. *See* Caregivers
    death cases, documentation, 223-224
    dynamics, 127
    indicators, 10t
    injuries, 18
    patterns, 9-21
        list, 10t
    physicians, tasks, 10t
    unfounded/uncharged allegations, investigation, 231
Abusive head injuries
    differentiation, unintentional, 9
    eye anatomy, relation, 107-111
    subdural hematoma, 102
Abusive head trauma (AHT), 2
    abuse patterns, 12-13
    autopsy, 191
        findings, 202-209
    biomechanics, 46-48
    cases, 249
    computer simulation program, usage (problems), 259
    education, 170-171
    findings, 113-116
    laboratory studies, 125t
    medical disorders, mimicking, 139
    mild, 12-13, 157t

N

O

P

Y

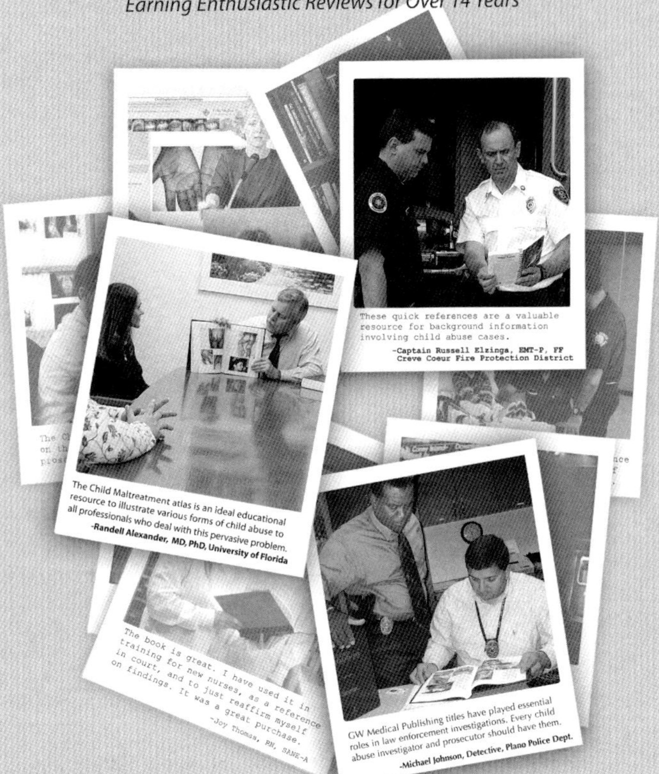

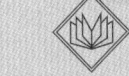

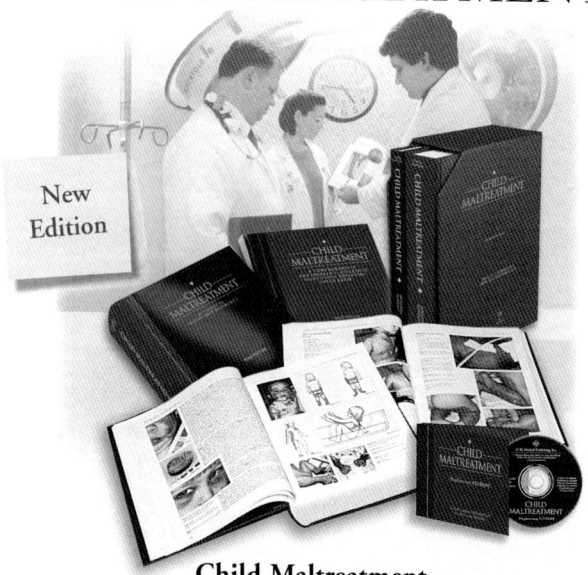

Quickly find digital images to help identify physical abuse

The *Child Maltreatment Supplementary CD-ROM* contains 300 full-color images with detailed case studies from field experts. All of the images are from our *Child Maltreatment Photographic Reference* and illustrate a diverse and comprehensive range of maltreatment and abuse circumstances. With the addition of a new slide presentation on physical abuse, this resource perfectly complements the 2-volume set for training presentations or self-study.

Contents

To order call toll-free **1-800-600-0330**

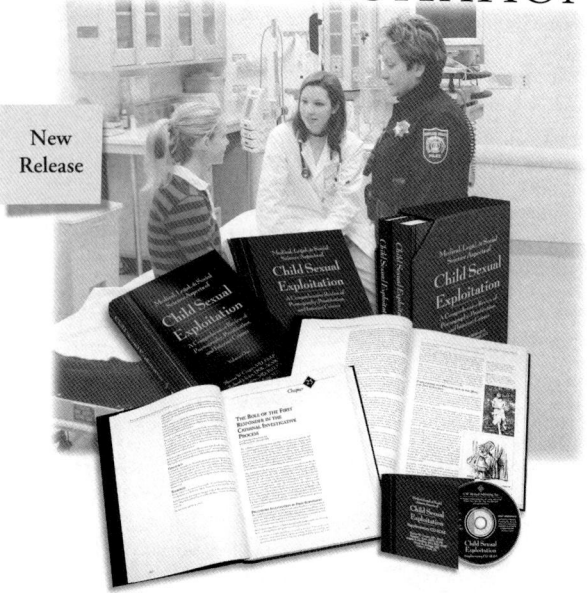

Addressing problems that arise from our global world, these books will be the standard for *law enforcement, medical, forensic, legal,* and *social science* professionals in the 21st century, empowering them to help stop this type of abuse.

Learn techniques used by lawbreakers in a multimedia environment

The *Child Sexual Exploitation Supplementary CD-ROM* is a researcher's companion to the 2-volume set. Users can learn how photos are circulated on the Internet and to spot digitally altered images. Users may also browse the extensive collection of more than 100 articles and government documents from the United States and abroad, assemble a collection of best practices from federal and local agencies, or create their own training curriculum using slide shows and case studies of sexual maturation, taxonomy of pornography, and sexually transmitted diseases.

Contents

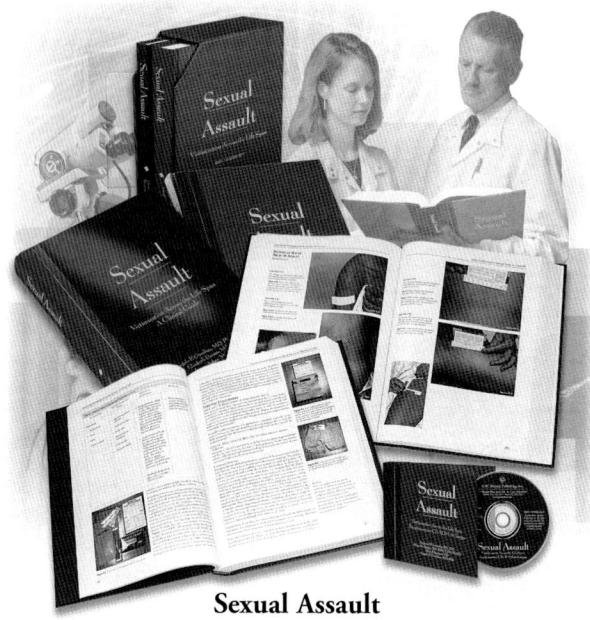

The *Sexual Assault Color Atlas* contains actual case studies from experts in the field, including more than 1400 high-quality clinical photos of sexually transmitted diseases, injuries in progressive stages of healing, and comparisons of injuries in multiple age groups. The atlas has special sections on victims with disabilities, assault during incarceration, cases involving DNA collection and analysis, and steps for prosecution.

The value of these two references cannot be overstated. Used together, they will aid professionals in dealing with sexual assault victims and lead the way to better evaluation and interpretation of their injuries.

Document and investigate sexual assault with the digital image library

The *Sexual Assault Supplementary CD-ROM* contains 130 full-color images with detailed case studies, all taken from the *Sexual Assault Color Atlas*, reflecting the findings that are most characteristic of the various age groups. The CD-ROM is a perfect complement to the 2-volume set, whether for training presentations or self-study.

Contents

To order call toll-free **1-800-600-0330**

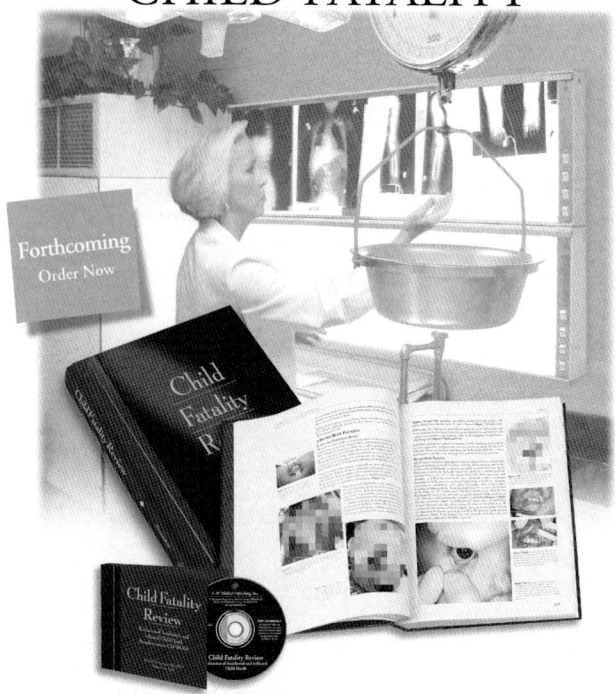

Case studies illustrate abusive and accidental forms of death, including neglect, SIDS, suicide, burning, drowning, and infectious diseases. This text is a powerful tool for all members of a child fatality review team and can guide anyone trying to form a new team.

While this illustrated text is an excellent tool for anyone who works on or with child fatality review teams, it is also an asset in the education arena. This reference is a valuable teaching tool in university social work classes or law enforcement teaching facilities.

Conveniently create presentations and test abilities with the CD-ROM

The *Child Fatality Review Supplementary CD-ROM* provides additional information to all professionals on these teams and allows members to test their abilities in reviewing difficult cases. It is a perfect complement to the text, whether for training presentations or self study.

Contents*

To order call toll-free **1-800-600-0330**

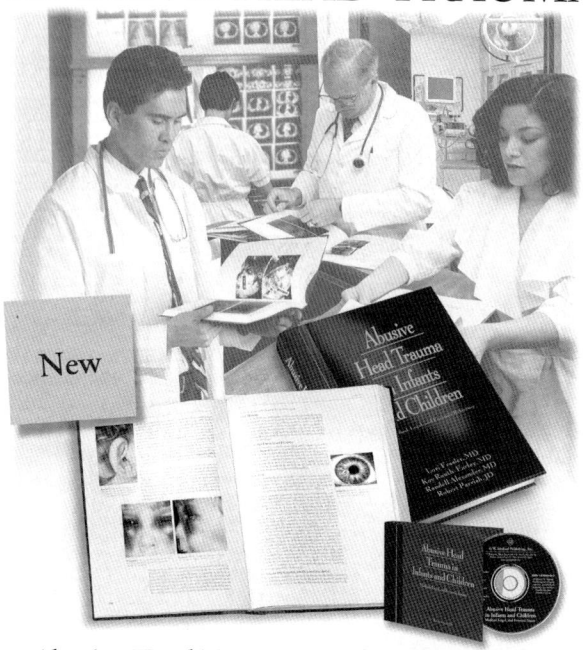

More than 600 clinical photos, case studies, and multidisciplinary analyses illustrate inflicted head injuries. Discussions of shaken baby syndrome, shaken impact syndrome, differential diagnoses, forensic analyses, autopsies, prosecutorial issues, long-term care of survivors, and the role of social services are featured.

This single-volume edition combines the best clinical writing with high-quality photographic content—a wealth of knowledge bound in one concise edition.

Show the reality of shaken baby syndrome with 3-D animations

The *Abusive Head Trauma Supplementary CD-ROM* uses 3-D images and animation developed from actual forensic analysis of victimized children to depict how head injuries occur. This product is valuable for explaining the complex biomechanics of abusive head injury to investigators and mandated reporters in an easy-to-understand format. Distinguish shaken baby syndrome from other types of head trauma with exacting animations developed by an esteemed pathologist.

Contents

CHILD SAFETY

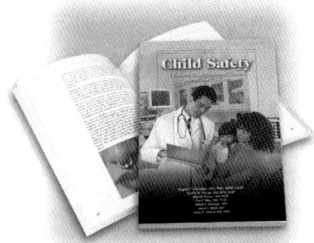

Child Safety
A Pediatric Guide for Parents,
Teachers, Nurses, and Caregivers

Protect children by helping them make wise decisions on their own

Child Safety addresses questions that arise throughout a child's development with discussions on topics ranging from child abuse to terrorism. Readers can easily access information using tables and checklists designed to highlight important issues.

This resource equips caregivers with the tools to protect their children and teach them to make wise decisions on their own.

Angelo P. Giardino, MD, PhD, MPH, FAAP;
Cynthia W. DeLago, MD, MPH, FAAP; Hans B. Kersten, MD, FAAP;
Paul S. Matz, MD, FAAP; Robert S. McGregor, MD; Laura E. Smals, MD;
Nancy D. Spector, MD, MPH

341 pages, 78 images, 9 contributors

Child Safety *ISBN 1-878060-67-8* $23.00

HELPING CHILDREN

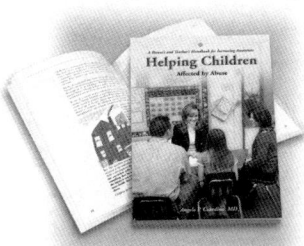

**Helping Children Affected
by Abuse**
A Parent's and Teacher's Handbook
for Increasing Awareness

Better understand child behavior and raise your awareness of abuse

Intended for parents, teachers, and caregivers, *Helping Children Affected by Abuse* will provide empowerment to protect children from abuse of any kind.

This book discusses physical, sexual, and emotional abuse and neglect, including warning signs and constructive responses for children. Stressing the importance of awareness, other topics discussed include nonabusive discipline, the dangers of the Internet, and the benefits of art therapy.

Angelo P. Giardino, MD, PhD, MPH, FAAP
218 pages, 51 images, 5 contributors

Helping Children Affected by Abuse *ISBN 1-878060-98-8* $23.00

To order or for more information, visit **www.gwmedical.com**